INTERMITTENT FASTING FOR WOMEN OVER 50

A Complete Guide to Losing Weight and Having a Healthier Lifestyle. Including 75 Recipes for Your Diet and Two 21-Day Meal Plans

Jenny Lee Brolin

© **Copyright 2021 by Jenny Lee Brolin - All rights reserved.**

The following Book is reproduced below with the goal of providing information that is as accurate and reliable as possible. Regardless, purchasing this Book can be seen as consent to the fact that both the publisher and the author of this book are in no way experts on the topics discussed within and that any recommendations or suggestions that are made herein are for entertainment purposes only. Professionals should be consulted as needed prior to undertaking any of the action endorsed herein.

This declaration is deemed fair and valid by both the American Bar Association and the Committee of Publishers Association and is legally binding throughout the United States.

Furthermore, the transmission, duplication, or reproduction of any of the following work including specific information will be considered an illegal act irrespective of if it is done electronically or in print. This extends to creating a secondary or tertiary copy of the work or a recorded copy and is only allowed with the express written consent from the Publisher. All additional right reserved.

The information in the following pages is broadly considered a truthful and accurate account of facts and as such, any inattention, use, or misuse of the information in question by the reader will render any resulting actions solely under their purview. There are no scenarios in which the publisher or the original author of this work can be in any fashion deemed liable for any hardship or damages that may befall them after undertaking information described herein.

Additionally, the information in the following pages is intended only for informational purposes and should thus be thought of as universal. As befitting its nature, it is presented without assurance regarding its prolonged validity or interim quality. Trademarks that are mentioned are done without written consent and can in no way be considered an endorsement from the trademark holder.

Table Of Contents

INTRODUCTION 6

CHAPTER 1: WHAT IS INTERMITTENT FASTING? 8
- What Is Intermittent Fasting? 8
- How Does IF Work? 8
- Why Does IF Work? 8
- What Effects Does It Have on Your Body Hormones? 9

CHAPTER 2: WHAT ARE THE EFFECTS OF INTERMITTENT FASTING ON METABOLISM? 12

CHAPTER 3: HOW INTERMITTENT FASTING HELPS THE BODY LOSE WEIGHT? 14
- What Is the Mechanism Behind Losing Weight? 14
- What Are the Barriers That Women Face When It Comes to Weight Loss? 15
- Relation Between Weight Loss and Intermittent Fasting 16

CHAPTER 4: HOW INTERMITTENT FASTING INCREASE YOUR ENERGY AND DETOX YOUR BODY? 18
- Can Fasting Give You More Energy? ... 18
- Ways of Detox Using Intermittent Fasting ... 19

CHAPTER 5: OTHER BENEFITS OF INTERMITTENT FASTING 22
- Lifestyle Benefits 22
- Health Benefits 22
- Cognitive Functioning Benefits 24

CHAPTER 6: WHAT IS AUTOPHAGY? 26
- Benefits of Autophagy 26

CHAPTER 7: COMMON MISTAKES DURING INTERMITTENT FASTING AND HOW TO AVOID THEM 30
- Pay Attention to Macronutrients 30
- Fat Is Not Bad 30
- Don't Get Greedy in the Feasting Windows ... 31
- Don't Try to Rush the Process 31
- Perseverance Is the Key 32
- Don't Frame Unrealistic Expectations ... 32
- Properly Manage Your Fasting Time ... 32

CHAPTER 8: ADVANTAGES AND DISADVANTAGES OF INTERMITTENT FASTING 34
- Advantages of Intermittent Fasting ... 34
- Disadvantages of Intermittent Fasting ... 35

CHAPTER 9: PATHOLOGIES AND CASES FOR WHICH INTERMITTENT FASTING IS NOT RECOMMENDED 38

CHAPTER 10: WHAT SIDE EFFECTS INTERMITTENT FASTING MIGHT HAVE 40
- Hunger 40
- Frequent Urination 41
- Headaches 41
- Cravings 41
- Heartburn, Bloating, and Constipation ... 42
- Binging 42
- Low Energy 42
- Feeling Cold 43

CHAPTER 11: HOW INTERMITTENT FASTING WILL HELP PEOPLE OVER 50 44
- How Intermittent Fasting Will Affect Women Over 50 Differently 44
- How Women Over 50 Can Benefit from Intermittent Fasting 44
- Nutrients You Need and How to Get Them ... 45

CHAPTER 12: WHAT HAPPENS AND WHAT ARE THE CHANGES IN THE HUMAN BODY WITH MENOPAUSE 48
- What Happens to the Body of a Menopausal Woman? 48
- The Ideal Diet for Menopause 49

CHAPTER 13: HOW INTERMITTENT FASTING CAN HELP AND MENOPAUSE WOMEN 52
- H 52
- ow to Use Intermittent Fasting in Your Menopause Stage? 52

CHAPTER 14: TYPES OF INTERMITTENT FASTING 56
- 5:2 and 4:3 Method 56
- 20/4 57
- Substituting Fasting 58
- 16/8 Daily Fasting 59
- The 1-Day Fast 59

CHAPTER 15: HOW TO INCLUDE AND ADAPT INTERMITTENT FASTING INTO YOUR LIFESTYLE 60

CHAPTER 16: FOOD LISTS 62
- Your Shopping List 62

Enjoy the Following Foods 63
Foods to Avoid 65

CHAPTER 17: INTERMITTENT FASTING AND OTHER DIETS 68

Difference with Ketogenic diet 69
Ketosis and Intermittent Fasting: The Physical Benefits 70

CHAPTER 18: THE RIGHT MINDSET TO FOLLOW THE DIET 72

Confide in Someone 72
Ensure You Are in a Conducive Environment .. 72
Support Groups 72
Seek Professional Help 73
Meditation and Positive Affirmations 73

CHAPTER 19: EXERCISES TO FEEL BETTER FOR WOMEN OVER 50 74

CHAPTER 20: 21-DAY (3-WEEKS) MEAL PLAN FOR 16/8 METHOD 76

CHAPTER 21: 21-DAY (3-WEEKS) MEAL PLAN FOR 5:2 METHOD 80

CHAPTER 22: BREAKFAST 84

1. Zucchini Omelet 84
2. Chili Omelet 85
3. Basil and Cherry Tomato Breakfast 86
4. Carrot Breakfast Salad 87
5. Garlic Zucchini Mix 88
6. Crustless Broccoli Sun-dried Tomato Quiche 89
7. Chocolate Pancakes 90
8. Breakfast Scramble 91
9. Oatmeal 92
10. Coconut Cream with Berries 93
11. Seafood Omelet 94
12. Spinach and Pork with Fried Eggs 95
13. Smoked Salmon Sandwich 96
14. Shrimp Deviled Eggs 97
15. Scrambled Eggs with Halloumi Cheese .. 98
16. Pancakes 99
17. Veggie Omelet 100
18. Ham Omelet 101
19. Savory Breakfast Muffins 102
20. Green Pineapple 103
21. Avocado Egg Bowls 104
22. Morning Meatloaf 105
23. Buttery Date Pancakes 106
24. Low Carb Pancake Crepes 107
25. Chia Seed Banana Blueberry Delight 108

CHAPTER 23: LUNCH 110

26. Cheesy Taco Skillet 110
27. Pork Chops with Mushroom Sauce 111
28. Beef Pot Roast 112
29. Creamy Southwest Chicken 113
30. Seafood Casserole 114
31. Shrimp Scampi 115
32. Seafood Soup 116
33. Crab Stuffed Mushrooms 117
34. Curried Tofu Scramble 118
35. Pesto Zucchini Spaghetti 119
36. Grilled Cauliflower Steak 120
37. Broccoli Fried Rice 121
38. Zucchini Green Bean soup 122
39. Mexican Cabbage Soup 123
40. Thai Shrimp Soup 124
41. Beef & Barley Soup 125
42. Instant Pot Chicken 126
43. Shrimp Salad 127
44. roccoli Salad 128
45. Southwest Chicken Salad 129
46. Tuna Salad 130
47. Black Bean & Quinoa Salad 131
48. Pasta Salad 132
49. Thai-Inspired Chicken Salad 133
50. Greek Quinoa Salad 134

CHAPTER 24: DINNER 136

51. Instant Pot Teriyaki Chicken 136
52. Teriyaki Salmon 137
53. Sheet Pan Steak Fajitas 138
54. Instant Pot Meatballs 139
55. Sheet Pan Chicken and Veggie Bake .. 140
56. Quinoa and Black Bean Casserole 141
57. Haddock with Spinach and Cauliflower Rice 142
58. Zoodles with White Clam Sauce 143
59. Creamy Lamb Korma 144
60. Fire-Roasted Tomato and Garlic Soup 145
61. Chicken and Prosciutto Spiedini 146
62. Pinchos de Pollo Marinated Grilled Chicken Kebabs 147
63. Slow Cooker Bacon and Chicken 148
64. Garlic Bacon Wrapped Chicken Bites 149
65. Smokey Bacon Chicken Meatballs 150
66. Asian Chicken Wings 151
67. Baked Garlic Ghee Chicken Breast ... 152
68. Crispy Chicken Thighs 153
69. Chicken and Bacon Sausages 154
70. Bifteck Hache (French Hamburgers) 155
71. Lemon Ghee Roast Chicken 156
72. Oven-Baked Parmesan Garlic Wings . 157
73. Crispy Indian Chicken Drumsticks ... 158
74. Whole Roast Chicken 159
75. Butternut Squash Tacos with Tempeh Chorizo 160

CONCLUSION 162

Introduction

Intermittent fasting is a good idea for women over 50. Intermittent fasting does not mean that you starve yourself. It just means that you do not eat every day and instead, will eat roughly every other day depending on your schedule and whether or not you are eating with a religious fast during that time. One way to make it work is to break the fast on Sundays when there most likely isn't going to be a religious obligation associated with it such as Catholic Mass or Ramadan. I also think that women over 50 may find intermittent fasting an easier way because they have more weight to lose than someone who is younger. This is the time when women are at their most vulnerable to begin losing muscle along with fat and this can easily lead to weight regain. It is much better for a woman over 50 to lose weight by fasting than it is for her to start an intense, very-low-calorie diet and risk muscle loss. When we lose weight slowly and gradually, our bodies will not perceive that as a sign of starvation but rather a reduction in caloric intake that can continue indefinitely.

Men do not have this problem because men don't lose as much muscle when they diet. They may lose some but they will gain the weight back more quickly than if they were women or if they had lost weight via intermittent fasting instead of crash diets.

Intermittent fasting, if it did not involve skipping any meals, would interfere with the circadian rhythm that comes with eating three meals a day at regular intervals. This is why women are advised to eat more frequently than men because men need less energy to sustain their bodies. This is why I think women over 50, or for that matter women of any age, may find this an easier way to lose weight. They don't have to starve themselves to do it but can instead modify the fasting schedule as they find their optimum pattern of modified fasting and then eating on a regular basis.

What is intermittent fasting? It is simply not eating for 12 hours at a time. You can do this either by skipping breakfast or eating a lighter dinner or both. Then you have to not eat again until the next day. Doing so results in weight loss and, as long as you are eating in moderation, will not cause muscle loss or other problems that you might find with other weight-loss regimens. This is because you are simply reducing calories from your usual intake so that it matches up better with your body's needs instead of forcing the body to get its necessary calories from fat cells, muscle, and other sources of energy when it doesn't need that energy.

I've seen intermittent fasting recommended for women over 50 in online articles and forums. Some of the articles refer to it as "eating normal." I know that skipping breakfast will also help me lose weight and keep it off even when I am not doing it on a regular schedule. I drink coffee without sweetener in the mornings but will skip breakfast if my schedule is tight or if I am not hungry in the morning for whatever reason. The same thing goes for dinner, too. If I eat a large lunch or dinner, I won't feel like eating again until lunchtime the following day.

CHAPTER 1:

What Is Intermittent Fasting?

What Is Intermittent Fasting?

IF isn't an eating routine, it's a way of eating. It's a method for booking your dinners so you benefit from them. It doesn't change what you eat, it changes when you eat. Indeed, more often than not you'll attempt to keep your calories similar when you start discontinuous fasting. (The vast majority eat greater suppers during a shorter time allotment.) Additionally, it is a decent method to keep bulk on while getting lean. With all that stated, the major reason individuals attempt this kind of fasting is to lose fat. This is an excellent thing since it implies discontinuous fasting falls into the class of "basic enough that you'll really do it, however significant enough that it will really have any kind of effect."

How Does IF Work?

To see how IF prompts fat misfortune we first need to comprehend the distinction between the fed state and the fasted state. Your body is in the fed state when it is processing and retaining nourishment. Regularly, the fed state begins when you start eating and goes on for three to five hours as your body processes and retains the nourishment you just ate. At the point when you are in the fed express, it's exceptionally difficult for your body to consume fat because your insulin levels are high. After that period, your body goes into what is known as the post-absorptive state, which is only an extravagant method for saying that your body isn't handling a feast. The post-absorptive state goes on until 8 to 12 hours after your last supper, which is the point at which you enter the fasted state. It is a lot simpler for your body to consume fat in the fasted state in light of the fact that your insulin levels are low. At the point when you're in the fasted express your body can consume fat that has been out of reach during the fed state. Since we don't enter the fasted state until 12 hours after our last supper, it's uncommon that our bodies are right now stated. This is one reason why numerous individuals who start discontinuous fasting will lose fat without changing what they eat, the amount they eat, or how regularly they work out. Fasting places your body in a fat-consuming state that you once in a while make it do, during a typical eating plan.

Why Does IF Work?

While IF might be a mainstream pattern in the eating regimen world nowadays, those attempting to get thinner or improve their general wellbeing should realize that it tends to be a hard arrangement to stick to. The methodology shifts back and forth between times of fasting and non-fasting during a specific timeframe.

IF isn't about hardship, however about separating your calories uniquely in contrast to the three-full dinners daily in addition to a nibble routine. The explanation IF is believed to be successful in weight reduction is on the grounds that it expands your body's responsiveness to insulin. Insulin, a hormone that is discharged when you eat nourishment, causes your liver, muscle and fat cells to store glucose. In a fasting state, blood glucose levels drop, which prompts a lessening in insulin creation, flagging your body to begin consuming put away vitality (starches). Following 12 hours of fasting, your body comes up short on put away vitality and starts consuming put away fat.

What Effects Does It Have on Your Body Hormones?

The advantages of IF are buzzing in the wellbeing scene with inquiring about supporting its capacity to decrease inflammation, heal the gut, and increment cell fix. While restricting nourishment admission for a while can do wonders for your wellbeing, there are a few concerns in regards to the potential symptoms it could have on hormonal wellbeing, particularly for those with thyroid issues, adrenal weakness, or other hormone uneven characters. So how about we jump profound into the hormone-fasting association with assistance decide whether this could be a decent mending device for you:

1. Fat putting away and hunger hormones: (leptin, insulin, + ghrelin)

Discontinuous fasting becomes the overwhelming focus in its job in improving yearning, digestion, and glucose influencing hormones. At the point when patients come in with blood sugar problems, it's good to prescribe IF because of its demonstrated capacity to increase metabolism and lower insulin obstruction. If you have a glucose issue and need to have a go at fasting, it's vital to work with your primary care physician who can screen you and easing back increment your length of fasting as your glucose stabilizes. Leptin opposition, another hormonal obstruction design that prompts weight put on and weight reduction obstruction, has likewise been appeared to improve with IF.

What's more, if you figure fasting would make you increasingly eager, reconsider. Irregular fasting has been appeared to emphatically influence the craving hormone ghrelin which can directly improve brain dopamine levels. This is the ideal case of the truth of the gut-mind pivot association.

2. Estrogen and progesterone

Your cerebrum and ovaries impart through the mind ovary hub or hypothalamic-pituitary-gonadal (HPG) pivot. Your cerebrum discharges hormones to your ovaries to flag them to discharge estrogen and progesterone. If your HPG hub isn't functioning admirably it can influence your general wellbeing and lead to issues with richness. With regards to IF, ladies are generally more delicate than men. This is due to the way women lose more leptin, which makes the effect on fasting more noticeable. If not done appropriately, IF can make ladies mess up their cycle and lose their hormones. While more research should be done it would bode well to legitimately reason that this hormonal move could influence digestion and richness as well.

Presently, this state since each individual is unique doesn't mean you can never attempt intermittent fasting. You may simply need to go at it with an alternate methodology. This fasting can be an incredible method to systematically bring fasting into your daily schedule.

3. Adrenal hormones (cortisol)

Cortisol is your body's fundamental pressure hormone and is discharged by your adrenal organs which sit directly on your kidneys. At the point when your mind adrenal (HPA) hub is lost, it can prompt awkwardness in cortisol. This high and low rollercoaster winds up driving to adrenal weakness. I've discovered that individuals with dysfunctions with their circadian beat don't deal with discontinuous fasting great. Nonetheless, attempting a moderate novice irregular fasting convention or the crescendo fasting could approve of somebody checking your advancement.

4. Thyroid hormones

Your thyroid is sovereign of all hormones influencing every cell in your body. No other hormone has that power. There is a wide range of types of thyroid problems all of which can be affected diversely by irregular fasting. Along these lines, it's good working with a useful medication professional who can work with your particular wellbeing case.

Plan of Intermittent Fasting, if you are:

Beginners
The 8-6 window plan: One simple way to IF is to just eat between 8 am and 6 pm. This allows for a long fasting period within a reasonable timeframe.
The 12-6 window plan: I personally do this plan during my workweek. This is the same as the last plan but extends the fast a couple more hours into lunchtime. I fill my morning with big cups of water and antioxidant-rich matcha tea.

Intermediate
Modified 2-day plan: Eat clean for five days and then restrict calorie intake to 700 on any two other days. Limited calorie intake can have similar effects as full fasting.
The 5-2 plan: Eat clean for five days and fully fast for two nonconsecutive days a week.

Advanced
Every-other-day plan: Fast fully every other day. While intense, it can be very effective for some people.

CHAPTER 2:

What Are the Effects of Intermittent Fasting on Metabolism?

RMR reveals the amount of energy or calories the body burns to survive without movement. In some places, this is calculated in BMR or basic metabolic price. RMR is responsible for approximately 70% of all your metabolism, so the final results listed here are impressive.

- Average RMR before cooking: 2,607 kcal burned/day
- Average RMR after 30 weeks in the program: 1,996 kcal burned/day
- Average RMR 6 years after final weighing: 1,903 kcal burned / day.

Despite the reality that participants returned about 70% of their first weight, their RMR did not return to pre-enrollment levels. It retained approximately 700 fewer calories per day! This indicates that to lose the same amount of weight in the second round, participants would need to eat 700 calories much less than the program. Because the initial diet contains 1200 to 1500 calories with 90 minutes of training 6 days a week. This would certainly be almost difficult. Why did RMR candidates continue to be so low even when they replaced the weight? The metabolic modification I have reviewed includes the BMR (basal metabolic rate) and also the RMR (resting metabolic price). Both explain how much energy (calories) your body uses to live without activity and represent approximately 70% of the entire metabolic process. This is not useful when the goal is permanent and lasting weight loss. Their results, once transformed, have remained stagnant and, in general, after the frustration that people offer and also all the accumulated weight, if they are lucky, their RMR/ BMR will improve. Weight gain, making sure to return to what you lose with a steady yo-yo diet, can result in a lower metabolic rate that will fight to lose weight and may even be the heaviest you have ever been. Therefore, if eating incorrectly causes this, you will most likely wonder exactly how you cannot improve your intake in any way for a long period. Keep reading to see why.

Comparison of intermittent fasting for low-calorie dietary strategies

Reduced calories do not create hormonal changes in the fasting agent. They are the trick to lose weight and also their redemption. Other hormones that I have not indicated for reasons of simplicity are also stimulated during this start window to stop metabolic rate reductions related to low-calorie diet strategies. Low-calorie diet plans still include consumption, and even every time we eat, blood sugar levels will increase, activating insulin.

Summary

- Low-calorie diet programs can ruin the metabolic procedure making sustainable weight loss almost impossible.
- Maintainable weight loss depends largely on the regulation of hormonal agents.
- Fasting prepares the main hormonal agents for metabolic retention, muscle retention, and weight loss.

Why should you try intermittent fasting?

There are excellent offers of various diet programs to choose from. Some help you limit your carbohydrate intake and concentrate on large fats and healthy proteins. Some will limit your fat intake and also focus on healthy, balanced, and excellent carbohydrates. With all the alternatives in the industry, at least some of them are reliable selections to lose weight, so you may wonder why you should choose intermittent fasting. This portion will analyze the various benefits of periodic fasting and also how you will distinguish your health.

It changes the characteristics of cells, hormones, and genetics

Numerous things happen in your body when you don't consume for a while. Your body will begin to initiate procedures for cell repair work, as well as to modify some of its hormone agent grades, which will facilitate access to maintained body fat. Other adjustments that may occur in the body include insulin grades: insulin levels will reach a reasonable level, making it easier for the body to melt fat. Blood levels of human development hormone can increase significantly. This can help build muscle tissue and burn fat. The body will certainly begin important mobile repair procedures, such as removing all debris from cells. Some useful changes in innumerable genes will help you live longer and also protect you from disease.

CHAPTER 3:

How Intermittent Fasting Helps the Body Lose Weight?

What Is the Mechanism Behind Losing Weight?

If you truly want to understand how you can lose weight or what makes you gain weight, then understanding certain hormonal functions is also important. Now, there are two very important hormones in your body that control the levels of blood glucose, and these are – insulin and glucagon. And there is another pair about whom you must have some knowledge and they are brown fat and white fat. You will keep gaining and losing weight and it is quite a natural fluctuation that the human body goes through. In order to understand this process, having full knowledge of these pairs is essential.

Insulin and Glucagon

You might have already done some research on how insulin is related to your blood glucose or blood sugar levels. But what we are going to discuss here is how any of this is related to gaining weight. Now, the place where insulin is made in your body is none other than the pancreas, and this insulin, in turn, is responsible for maintaining proper levels of blood glucose.

People suffer from hyperglycemia when the levels of glucose in their blood become high. Similarly, they suffer from hypoglycemia when the levels of glucose in their blood become low. When you are eating food, there is a subsequent rise in the levels of glucose in your blood. This is because the food is being digested as a result of which glucose is formed by the transformation of carbohydrates. This glucose is then utilized by the organ systems so that they can get the energy to perform their activities. Now, when you think about carbs, I bet that the first food items that come to your mind are probably something along the lines of pasta and bread, but there are so many veggies and fruits that are rich in carbs as well.

Now, when there is a rise in the levels of glucose in the blood, insulin is released from the pancreas. The task of insulin is to signal the fats, muscles, and liver in your body to start the absorption of glucose from the bloodstream. This is the actual process in which the different organ systems derive energy. When the amount of glucose is more in the blood than what is actually required, the glucose gets stored in the form of glycogen in the liver. Sometimes, insulin helps in converting excess glucose into fatty acids. The adipose tissues in your body are where the fats are stored.

Now, there are three things that are inhibited by the presence of insulin, and they are as follows – gluconeogenesis, glycogenolysis, and lipolysis. So, lipolysis is when your body engages in the breakdown of fats in order to derive energy for day-to-day activities. Glycogenolysis is when usable glucose is formed by the breakdown of glycogen. The process is inhibited by the presence of insulin. And lastly, gluconeogenesis is when the non-carbohydrate sources act as the substrate from which glucose is created.

So, we have two hormones working behind the scenes. The three mechanisms mentioned above are set into motion by the presence of glucagon, and these mechanisms are the reason why there is a rise in the levels of glucose in your blood. But the presence of insulin has the capability of inhibiting these mechanisms and then reducing the levels of glucose in the blood.

What Are the Barriers That Women Face When It Comes to Weight Loss?

There was a study that was conducted by the Yale Journal of Biology and Medicine, and in it, it was stated how women are more prone to being obese than men. In fact, the chances of a woman being obese are twice that of a man. Now, if you are wondering why then here are the reasons –

Hormones

One of the biggest reasons for women being more prone to weight gain is their hormonal makeup. Factors like diet, aging, and stress play a big role in the alteration of hormones like estrogen, cortisol, and progesterone, and obesity is a by-product of all these changes taken together. The reason behind women not being adapted to these hormonal changes is because our diets are being increasingly composed of foods that are highly processed.

Also, the process of storing fat in the body of a woman is influenced by the hormone estrogen, which is also known as the female sex hormone. One of the most common signs of aging in women is that they start gaining weight and losing muscles and the major reason is the reduction in the level of estrogen. An important event in the life of women over the age of 50 is menopause and with menopause comes the reduction of estrogen in the body.

Metabolism

The process of metabolism that is present in women is not the same as that in men, and there are some differences that will show you how it acts as a barrier to weight loss. The amount of lean muscles is more in men than in women and this greater number of lean muscles is one of the reasons why the resting metabolic rate of men is higher. There is a scientific reason behind it too. The efficiency of muscles to burn calories is much more than fats. So, possessing a greater number of lean muscles automatically means that they are going to burn more calories. Therefore, even if a man does not engage in any strenuous physical activity, he will consume more calories than a woman doing the same thing.

The process becomes worse because of the fact that the storage of fat is also different between the two genders. The fat, in the case of women, is mostly stored in areas like thighs, buttocks, and hips. And any fitness expert can confirm that these are exactly the regions which need a lot of effort to shed fat from.

Emotions

Yes, no matter how you feel about this one but emotions do play a big role when it comes to weight loss, especially in women. The American Journal of Clinical Nutrition confirms the fact that emotional eating is something that women are more engaging with than men. It was in the year 2013 that this study was published.

Some of the findings that this research had are as follows –
- Women are more inclined towards maintaining a diet, but maintaining something consistently for a period of time also requires an immense amount of motivation and willpower. Both these factors can be adversely affected by fluctuation in emotions that can, in turn, lead to stress. Also, it was found that emotional eating was a case that was more common in those women who were following some kind of diet and not that much common in those who were not following any diet at all. Thus, women need to be more aware of the factors that can cause stress and trigger an emotional eating response.
- Probably the worst part about someone engaging in emotional eating is that they will not go for a healthy smoothie or kale salad in case something is bothering them, or they are utterly depressed. Instead, they will reach out for sugary stuff like ice cream, cookies, and chocolates, all of whom have a lot of calories.
- Lastly, it is not that much to break out of a pattern of emotional eating. But at the end of the day, emotional eating is nothing but a learned behavior, and such behaviors can be unlearnt with proper effort and willpower. But you have to realize that you are in this vicious cycle and you have to break free otherwise if you go too deep into it, then breaking free will become equally difficult.

Genetics

The genetic makeup of a person is also one of the reasons why they are more prone to obesity than others. For example, if every woman in your lineage had a tendency to be over the average BMI, then there are high chances that you will have the same tendency too. So, no matter how much effort you put into weight loss, these factors will still be working against you.

So, the only thing that you have to do is keep reminding yourself not to expect any results soon. In order to lower your BMI, one of the key steps to take is to live an incremental lifestyle. But yes, intermittent fasting definitely is an effective tool to help you in your weight loss journey.

Relation Between Weight Loss and Intermittent Fasting

Now that we are talking about fat and glucose and the difference between them as energy sources, you must have understood that even fat is just the way the body stores energy. In order to make fat more easily available to your body, there are certain changes taking place in your body during the fasting window. These are all related to the metabolism of the body, and they are explained below –
- Insulin Levels – The level of insulin in the human body shows an increase whenever you are eating something. In the same manner, the opposite happens when you do not eat food; that is, the level of insulin decreases. And when this happens, the process of fat burning is facilitated.
- Human Growth Hormone or HGH – The levels of this hormone increase to five or six times their usual amount during the fasting window. The main functions of this hormone include loss of fat and gain in muscles, but apart from this, it helps in a lot of other things as well.
- Norepinephrine – The fat cells receive norepinephrine when you are on a fast as a message sent by the nervous system. After this, the formation of fatty acids takes place in the body. Then, they serve as an alternative source of fuel to cater to your body's energy requirements.

A fasting period of about forty-eight hours can really boost your body's metabolic rate by as much as 3.6-14%, and this was published in The American Journal of Physiology. But similarly, if you do not want your metabolic rates to go off the rails and show drastic reduction instead, then you need to keep fasting periods under control.

The process of weight loss happens merely through a deficit of calories, and that is exactly what happens when you engage in intermittent fasting. Since you are skipping meals, you are reducing your calorie intake. This does not depend on the method of intermittent fasting you are following. No matter what method you follow, you will still be reducing your calories. But there is also something else to keep in mind here. When you are in your eating window, you have to limit your calorie consumption and not overdo it because if you eat too much, there will no longer be any calorie deficit and your fasting will not bring any results.

The ways in which intermittent fasting helps your body to lose weight are as follows –

- Reduction in Stored Fat – During the fasting window, both the amounts of glucose and glycogen are depleted so fast, and so insulin sensitivity improves after a certain period of time. This means that your body gradually becomes used to utilizing lower insulin amounts as a result of a reduced blood sugar level. Also, the efficiency of utilization of glucose also improves. Moreover, since the amount of insulin present in your blood in the fasting period is limited, the blood sugar is also not able to reach any other areas than where it is supposed to. So, it does not get added to the fat storage of your body. Thus, the amount of fat that you have already lost will not be regained.

CHAPTER 4:

How Intermittent Fasting Increase Your Energy and Detox Your Body?

Can Fasting Give You More Energy?

Intermittent fasting, as high as it sounds, is not for everyone. Think of it as a new lifestyle for which the body needs to adapt first. It's normal at first to experience a loss of energy, extreme hunger, and even dizziness. The benefits only show up after a couple of weeks. So be careful, and don't base your opinion on your initial feeling. Stick in there and allow your body to acclimatize to its new lifestyle. Overtime will decrease the production of the hormone ghrelin that influences your sense of hunger and satiety, making you less hungry and more energetic.

We may already have some understanding of the effects of what we eat in terms of our food quality and quantity, but have we stopped considering the impact of when we eat it? Why everyone is told that breakfast is the most important meal of the day and that we should eat all day long from 8 a.m. to 8 p.m. for energy? Is that "first meal" really a need to have in the morning, and could it be likely that missing a meal can be beneficial? Join intermittent fasting, an eating style that shortens the period individual eats and increases the period that an individual fasts. Remember that while there are different approaches for doing intermittent fasting, I will concentrate on convenience on the "skip breakfast" approach.

So how is one slipping into sporadic fasts? The quick and straightforward answer is not to eat breakfast and continue the first lunch meal. Further, Black coffee, tea, and water are fine to drink at lunchtime, respectively. When you finally break your fast, your lunch content doesn't have to be anything else-a standard lunch is perfectly fine (unless you have a specific diet plan or goals that you need to meet). Also, your dinner portion is the same when it's time for that (unless you have other projects), but note the hour you're eating the dinner. The period of fasting begins from the time you finish dinner to the time you eat lunch again— the period you sleep included. So, on paper, the intermittent fasting periods can be written as [period fasting/period eating], where 18/6 IF tends to be a very soft sweet spot when taking into account the busy lifestyle of a person. 16/8 is a bit easier, but 20/4 or even 22/2 comes with even more satisfying benefits if you can.

Before I get into the explanation of the mechanisms of what happens to the body when you're fasting, take a second to think about the benefits of shifting to having only two meals that may already result. If all meals are about the same size, eating less through fasting is equivalent to spending less time preparing, less money buying food and less stress on worrying about what to eat. A lower calorie consumption comes with that, and (to some extent) caloric restriction is equivalent to weight loss. (For those who try to gain weight, eating more substantial portions with a proper distribution of macronutrients will balance it out.) The gist of intermittent fasting is that you look good and feel good, but now why would that be?

Our body is filled with hormones, and many of them play a role in controlling our energy balance so that the hunger-and satiety-related signals are essential and timed accordingly. Signaling pathway impairments, such as aberrant expression of a hormone, may lead to a variety of health problems and neurodegenerative diseases, including obesity, CVD, hypertension, diabetes, and Alzheimer's. Leptin and insulin are the two leading players who are related to energy balance. Leptin is secreted from fat cells in a proportional amount to an individual's amount of adipose tissue, which acts with insulin to serve as an appetite suppressant signal effectively. The main functions of insulin are to facilitate the absorption of glucose from food into the body and also to encourage energy storage in the form of liver muscle and adipose tissue. Upon insulin release and increased fat stores, food consumption results, but what if you didn't want to hold on to those fat stores? In this situation, intermittent fasting is the logical answer. As you stop eating for a while longer, the insulin level of your body is low and compensates for the deficit by increasing lipolysis so that your fat stores are used for energy.

Ways of Detox Using Intermittent Fasting

You cringe when you hear the word "fast," imagining ten consecutive days consuming nothing but lemon juice, a maple syrup, and cayenne pepper mixture that you've listened to celebrities use for extreme weight reduction?

Yet, do you fear that the end of this great deprivation will only lead to a rapid recovery of all weight, a decrease in metabolism, constipation, or even severe illness such as problems with the gallbladder? Further, put your mind at ease in knowing that intermittent fasting that has gained popularity since 2012 is a healthier, more realistic, and more sustainable alternative to traditional continuous 2 to 10-day fasts. Physicians, scientists, and writers have, in fact, strongly supported various forms of detox with intermittent fasting, of which 11 are listed below:

Skipping Breakfast

This intermittent form of fasting lasts from 8 p.m. By 12-noon challenges the theory that Breakfast is the most important meal of the day. Now the three-meal-a-day tradition that began in Europe in the 1600s. Nutritional expert and author of the book Glow15, Naomi Whittel, demonstrates that skipping Breakfast stimulates autophagy or cellular regeneration, removing harmful cell waste, strengthening the immune system, and reducing inflammation. (10) The American Society of Nutrition's 16-fold clinical trial in 2014 found that neither eating nor skipping Breakfast affected weight loss.

Eating Only When Skipping Hungry / Spontaneous Meal
Wait to Live, do not love to eat, as described. It negates binging's emotional eating habits when excited or sad, which leads to weight gain. Skipping spontaneous meals is good for the body and adapted individually, making it highly sustainable. You choose to eat within any timeframe your body is signaling and never be obligated to eat on the terms of someone else.

The 12:12

Fast Recommended for intermittent fasting beginners; this detox form involves eating during a 12-hour window followed by 12-hour fasting. Studies have found that fat transfer occurs within 10 to 16 hours of fasting. This quick let you eat three meals plus one balanced, light snack that can be spread out every three hours. Remember that feeding every three hours cuts off the protection mechanism for starvation (which in turn promotes the burning of abdominal fat by the cortisol hormone), retains lean muscle tissue, and revives the metabolism.

The 5-Day Mini-Fast
It is created by nutritionist Kellyann Petrucci and featured on a Dr. Oz episode, the 15:2 Mini-Fast, which involves eating a personalized diet from 11 a.m. for eight hours. And 7:00 p.m. Over a duration of 5 days. The layout of this diet is as follows:
- Breakfast: liquid such as a slimming shake with berries, protein, and greens; coffee; tea; or one lemon juice tablespoon in eight ounces of water.
- Lunch: A fat-burning meal of 4 ounces of protein and 2 ounces of healthy fat.
- Dinner: Includes 4 ounces of protein, 2 ounces of healthy fat, and 1/2 cup of cooked beans.
- Dessert: almond milk, avocado, cocoa powder, few drops of coconut oil, and vanilla extract.

The 16:8 fast or Leangains diet
It focuses more on time measurement than calorie measurement. This involves eating during an eight-hour window followed by fasting for women up to 14 hours and for men 16 hours and is usually done every other day. Further, a six-week study, published in the World Journal of Diabetes, was conducted in which participants with type 2 diabetes normally ate on weeks one to two and five to six, while fasting (including skipping Breakfast) was conducted on weeks three to four with an 18 to 20-hour daily fasting target, drinking only tea or coffee. This study produced results of intermittent, morning fasting correlated with at-target blood glucose levels, and weight loss.

The idea behind the ability of fasting to treat diabetes concludes that, during fasting, fat cells release stored sugar that is converted into energy, resulting in a decrease in insulin levels and weight loss. (7) VIII. The 20:4 Fast / Warrior Diet This intermittent fasting approach is inspired by the tribal eating system, where hunting took place all day, accompanied by one meal at night. Moreover, it consists of raw fruits and vegetables during a 20-hour fast, leaving room for one big dinner, during a 4-hour period that includes carbohydrates, protein, plenty of vegetables, and healthy fats. While the warrior diet appeals to tonight eaters, it is not for everyone as digesting large meals before bedtime burdens the digestive system. You may argue that this diet allows portion control of binge eating and sabotage.

The 5:2 Fast
This detox approach involves five days of ordinary eating, followed by two days of very limited calorie use (maximum 500 calories for women or 600 calories for men). The two days of fasting are often spread out in between, with at least one day. Further, The International Journal of Obesity reports a six-month study that was conducted among 107 obese and overweight women aged 30 to 45 years to compare continuous fasting (two days) with intermittent fasting (seven days). Participants in the fasting days ate 25 percent of their calorie needs. The study results showed that the benefits of intermittent fasting mirrored that of continuous fasting when it came to weight loss, and the benefits of intermittent fasting for disease prevention exceeded that of continuous fasting due to increased tolerance to cellular stress.

Several-Day Juice
Dr. Joel Fuhrman, author of the book Fasting and Eating for Health, states that juicing works by reducing the calories and decreasing the toxic load found in processed foods, which gives the body more energy to regenerate, thus increasing its lifespan. The juice is preferred over water, as it contains nutrients that are vital to the removal of toxins and contains electrolytes that

prevent discharge. During this fast, Dr. Fuhrman recommends vegetable juices plus one salad a day. A sample quicking juice would contain one fruit serving combined with various other vegetables such as carrots, cabbage, kale, beets, and cucumbers. Furthermore, Every-Other-Day Fast This fast, achieved on alternating days, ranges from being abstained from solid foods to reducing calories to 500 and then eating unlimited calories on feeding days. The Nutritional Journal conducted a 12-week study of 32 average and obese people, alternating a fast day with a feed day (consumption of 25 percent of caloric needs). The results showed weight loss and heat gain with alternate-day fasting. During the 12-week period, the participants lost more than 11 pounds.

24-Hour Once-A-Week Fast

This is a fast done once a week from breakfast to breakfast, lunch-to-lunch, or dinner-to-dinner, allowing for non-caloric beverages like herbal tea. Only after mastering a 12-hour fast is a word of advice to progress to a 24 hour fast. Further, you can prepare for this type of fast by eating a low-carbohydrate, three-month, nutrient-rich diet that stabilizes insulin and lessens the feeling of hunger.

CHAPTER 5:

Other Benefits of Intermittent Fasting

Lifestyle Benefits

When compared to other diets, the simplicity of intermittent fasting makes it perhaps the easiest eating protocol through which to experience significant health benefits. Often, the complexity of some eating plans causes people to fail at the first hurdle because as much as they think they understand what they should be doing, they really don't. This results in people going to punishing extremes in order to fulfill what they think they are supposed to be doing and ending up with very disappointing results. Intermittent fasting couldn't be simpler—now you eat and now you don't. Often, special diets can be extremely expensive to follow. You have to purchase special ingredients and eat food that you ordinarily wouldn't. Intermittent fasting is different in that regard too. It costs you absolutely nothing to practice intermittent fasting, and other than a caloric reduction in the case of weight loss and eating as healthy as possible, there is no dictation as to what to eat.

Intermittent fasting is flexible, so it allows you gaps in between to eat the things you enjoy. What is life without an occasional dessert, some chocolate, or pizza? With intermittent fasting, you can have those treats and not feel guilty because when you fast, your body will be burning that treat off. Of course, that is not to say that in every eating window you can binge on every fast food known to mankind. You will still need to eat a healthy diet; you just won't be weighing food and calculating its calorie content all the time.

If you have found an eating plan that you enjoy such as Keto, Paleo, or the like, you can incorporate that with intermittent fasting. There are no other plans available where you can combine two and get even better results. Intermittent fasting is a fantastic addition to other eating plans and does not detract from any other diets (Fung, 2020).

For women over 50, the adjustment to menopause can mean a temporary change in lifestyle. In severe situations, menopause can result in difficulties in relationships with partners and loved ones. Intermittent fasting can help make a big difference in these challenges, and this can be life-changing.

Health Benefits

Cardiovascular health should be a strong focus for people of all ages but even more so for women over 50. The most significant cause of death for women over 50 today is cardiovascular disease. This umbrella term describes all diseases of the heart or the arteries leading to and from the heart. This could include blockages, damage, and deformities in the structure. There are several risk factors that contribute to the occurrence of cardiovascular disease including smoking, physical inactivity, genetics, and diet. The latter, however, has been found to be the largest controllable contributor to heart disease.

The most impactful factor where diet is concerned is the types of protein sources that are eaten as well as the types of fats that are consumed. Plant proteins such as beans and legumes have been proven to be a healthier source of protein than animal proteins in general.

Where animal protein is concerned, the leaner the source, the better, and poultry and fish are always healthier options than red meat. The fat component of red meat is another problem where heart disease is concerned, as are other sources of fat such as cooking oils and spreads used for bread. Saturated fats are the types of fats we want to avoid in our diet, and these include animal fat, lard, and tropical oils such as palm oil. Unsaturated fats in small quantities are healthier. Examples of unsaturated fats include avocados, nuts, olive oil, and vegetable oils. When we eat foods in excess of what our body is able to burn, the leftover food forms triglycerides that, at high levels, contribute to the occurrence of cardiovascular disease. When we fast, our body burns triglycerides for energy thereby reducing the levels in our blood and, in turn, reducing our risk of cardiovascular disease.

In the last chapter, we discussed the impact of intermittent fasting on insulin levels. In our eating window, we experience an increase in insulin levels, and when we fast, those levels are decreased. This decrease in insulin results in less food being stored as fat. In animal trials, intermittent fasting has been shown to prevent and reverse Type 2 Diabetes. Another thing that happens when insulin levels decrease is that the FOXO transcription factors, which are known to positively impact metabolism, become more active in the body. This process is also linked to improved longevity and healthy aging.

Another non-communicable disease that seems to be impacted by intermittent fasting is cancer. Growth Factor 1 (GF1) is a hormone very similar in nature to insulin, and the presence of this hormone is known to be a marker for cancer development. Levels of GF1 are reduced during intermittent fasting. Women over 50 are twice as likely to develop breast cancer, for instance, and risk factors for other common cancers are also thought to increase when women start to experience the hormonal changes of menopause. Intermittent fasting is, therefore, an excellent preventative measure for the occurrence of cancer in women over 50.

The increased cell resilience is seen in people who regularly fast has been linked to a stronger immune system as well as a general faster recovery from illness. The process of building cell resilience through fasting is similar to exercising muscles. The more you undertake regular exercise with periods of rest in between, the stronger your muscles become.

The autophagy process that is triggered by intermittent fasting has been shown to help reduce inflammation in the body as well as oxidative stress, which is primarily responsible for cell damage in the body. Inflammation in various parts of the body has been shown to be present as a precursor to the diagnosis of many different non-communicable diseases. The diagnosis of non-communicable diseases is far more common in women over 50 than any other age group. It is, therefore, vital for women in this age group to make use of intermittent fasting and autophagy as an additional preventative measure against the development of non-communicable diseases.

The Circadian Cycle is the name given to the rhythm created in our body by light and dark (day and night). This natural rhythm controls our need to sleep and eat and has a major impact on our metabolism, cognitive function, and emotional health. It is our internal clock, and when disrupted, it can have devastating effects on our bodies. Intermittent fasting has been shown to help regulate the Circadian Cycle and, if it is out of the loop, reset it back to its natural function.

From an evolutionary perspective, our bodies are designed to eat during the day and not to eat at night. This, of course, is the reverse in certain nocturnal mammals who have evolved to reverse that Circadian Cycle due to the availability of prey at night. As modern humans, we have disrupted our Circadian Cycle by not going to sleep when the sun goes down and also continuing to eat well into the night. This impacts our metabolism and our sleeping patterns, resulting in weight gain and sleep disorders such as insomnia. By using intermittent fasting to reset our internal clock to its evolutionary default, we can encourage weight loss by optimizing our metabolism and have a more restful sleep.

In women over 50, this is particularly beneficial. As we age, sleep disorders become more common. We feel tired earlier, experience disturbed sleep, and generally find that we are unable to sleep for as many hours as we once could. This disruption in sleep, of course, has a major impact on our health both physically and mentally. The reason for this change in sleep is due to the reduced levels of Human Growth Hormone (HGH) in our bodies as we age. As we now know, intermittent fasting helps to increase the levels of HGH in our body, thus allowing us to regain a more regular sleeping pattern.

It is important to point out that your last meal of the day should be eaten at least two hours before you go to sleep, and it should be a satisfying but not overly large meal. If you eat too long before you go to bed, you may experience hunger pangs while you sleep that disrupt your sleep. If you eat too large a meal before going to sleep, your body will still be diverting additional blood flow to your stomach to digest its contents, and that will also disrupt your sleep. The importance of a good sleeping pattern cannot be understated as poor sleeping patterns have even been shown to increase the likelihood of the occurrence of certain cancers.

Intermittent fasting has also been shown to improve the regulation of genes that promote liver health and also in the balance of gut bacteria. Gut bacteria play a role in our immune system, and it is vital to keep these gut guests in good shape to optimize your body's defense systems (Kresser, 2019).

Cognitive Functioning Benefits

As you move into your 50s, there are several different effects on your brain health and, as a result, on your cognitive functioning. Brain shrinkage automatically occurs as we age, and although it is not something we can avoid, it is certainly something that we can delay and slow down. From a fasting perspective, the process of autophagy, which speeds up during fasting, can help to consume damaged brain cells and use that cellular material to produce new brain cells. This process can help to alleviate the natural brain shrinkage process.

The release of ketones during the burning of fat which occurs during fasting is also highly beneficial to brain health. The enhanced level of ketones helps to protect the brain from the development of epileptic seizures, Alzheimer's Disease and other neurodegenerative diseases. Of course, as we age, we are also more likely to develop neurodegenerative diseases. Diseases like Alzheimer's and other forms of dementia do have a wide range of risk factors including genetics and smoking. Fasting to enhance autophagy and ketone production is one way that we put up a line of defense against these diseases.

A study conducted on participants over 50, all of whom were already exhibiting some form of impaired cognitive function, showed that by increasing the levels of ketones in the participants' bodies, their cognitive functioning increased within six weeks. It is believed that the reason ketones are so beneficial in increasing cognitive function is due to the fact that they trigger the release of brain-derived neurotrophic factor (BDNF). BDNF helps to strengthen the neural connections in our brain, which are the pathways that our brain uses to transmit thoughts and instructions. BDNF particularly helps to strengthen the pathways that focus on memory and learning. Studies have also shown that intermittent fasting also helps to promote the growth of new nerve cells in the brain.

Intermittent fasting can also help to improve neuroplasticity, which is the brain's natural capability to build new neural pathways. This is imperative in learning as well as in the breaking of habits.

When we break bad habits, we actually work to remove the brain's reliance on a commonly used neural pathway and promote the use of a new pathway. Studies in people with brain injuries have shown that intermittent fasting speeds up healing.

CHAPTER 6:

What Is Autophagy?

Fasting has been found to stimulate a bodily process called autophagy. Autophagy is the metabolic process by which the body breaks down old, damaged cells and abnormally developing cells. The term autophagy is derived from the Greek words "auto" ("self") and "phagy" ("eating"), and translates to "self-eating." It is the way in which your body consumes your tissues and renews your cellular processes.

Autophagy is the human body's system for cleansing itself; it is like an internal recycling program. It is your built-in mechanism for getting rid of old cells and recycling your damaged parts for energy. It is how you get rid of your unhealthy or impaired parts and create younger, healthier cells. Autophagy is a very carefully controlled process that makes your bodily systems, organs, and processes more efficient. It helps clear waste and cells that you no longer need from your body.

Autophagy is the body's response to stressful or unfamiliar environments. Autophagy kicks in when it needs to, helping to defend your body against the negative effects of stress. It is your body's way of protecting itself, slowing the aging process, and promoting longevity.

When cells no longer work well or are damaged, they need to be removed from the body so that they do not multiply. If they are not removed from the body, they can block pathways and contribute to the cause of disease. If damaged or dysfunctional cells are allowed to accumulate, they will either die or become cancerous.

The accumulation of old, damaged cells may contribute to the aging process and the development of the disease. Both Alzheimer's disease and several types of cancer have been linked to having old, damaged proteins accumulating in the body. The process of clearing out old proteins may thus prevent the development of such diseases. In the brain, when not enough autophagy takes place, the result may be neurodegeneration or dysfunction within the brain. It is thus imperative that the body is regularly given a chance to find and destroy those cells that have gone wrong. This may lower the overall risk of developing the disease.

Benefits of Autophagy

Autophagy is critical in not only protecting the body from disease, but also for slowing down the aging process and promoting general health and well-being. The process of autophagy benefits the nervous system, the immune system, the heart, as well as your metabolism. It also plays a part in improving cognitive function by encouraging the growth of brain cells and nerve cells. Autophagy promotes a high-performing, body, and brain.

Inflammation

A great number of health conditions have been linked to chronic inflammation. Inflammation occurs naturally in all parts of the body, it is how your body responses to stress, and to the pathogens and toxins that try to infect it. Eating an unhealthy diet, lack of exercise, poor lifestyle choices and prolonged stress can all lead to issues with immune response. Overactive immune systems or chronic inflammation can cause intestinal problems, heart disease, diabetes, cancer, and various neurodegenerative diseases. Many people have issues with chronic inflammation without even realizing it. Symptoms can be quite subtle and longstanding, but many will get worse over time.

The process of autophagy plays a part in controlling inflammation in your body and increasing your immunity towards disease. It promotes just the right amount of inflammation that the body needs to be healthy and keeps the immune response where it needs to be.

Autophagy increases inflammation in the body when you need to fight something off, and decreases inflammation when you need it less. When there is an intruder to the body, autophagy encourages the signals that cause inflammation and increases the natural killer cells that you need to fight the infection or disease. It turns on the immune response to prevent the intruder from attacking the body. The same process then decreases inflammation when it is no longer needed by clearing the cells that stimulate the immune response once the threat is gone.

Autophagy has been shown to be beneficial in fighting inflammatory diseases such as Crohn's disease, arthritis, and cystic fibrosis.

Fighting Disease
The systems within your body constantly burn fuel or fat for energy. As this process occurs, dangerous toxins can build up in your body and damage your cells. In order to keep your cells in good, healthy condition, you must break down these toxins proactively before they can do any damage. Healthy cells work more efficiently than partially damaged ones do.

Autophagy allows for this cleansing process to happen. It helps fight disease in some very specific ways. Autophagy removes damaged parts of cells, removes toxins created by infection, and modulates the body's immune response to infection.

Muscle Performance
Autophagy prevents damage to your healthy tissues and organs and makes your muscle cells stronger and more resistant to wear and tear.

Working out causes microscopic tears in your muscles, which leads to some inflammation. After exercise, your muscles are worn out and require repair. They respond to this stress by going through autophagy. This is when your body will go to work to break down the damaged components of your muscles in order to rebuild them. Autophagy repairs the microscopic damage that you caused during the workout. This process of repair is what leads your muscles to grow and strengthen. Each time they go through autophagy, muscles get a little bigger and a little stronger. This is why experts will tell you that it is important for you to give your body time to recover in between workouts. You need time to reap the full benefits of autophagy.

Autophagy also keeps your energy expenditures in check. Your body's goal is to reduce the amount of energy required by your muscles. It does this by recycling as much existing energy as it can.

Digestive Health
Digestion is a process that occurs in the gastrointestinal tract by which food is converted into other substances that the body can use. Every time you eat food, the cells in your gastrointestinal tract work on overdrive so that you can digest the food. Autophagy gives these cells a chance to repair and restore themselves. They are removed from any stacks that have occurred and are given a chance to heal from any damage that has occurred.

Autophagy is critical to gut health. It gives your entire digestive system a much-needed break, allowing your body to focus on both saving energy and healing itself. Autophagy in your intestinal lining makes you less susceptible to gut inflammation as well as the formation of the leaky gut syndrome.

Brain

Autophagy may provide protection against the development of psychiatric issues and disorders related to the brain. Disruptions to autophagy have been linked to an increased risk of psychiatric problems. Scientific investigation into the brains of individuals with depression and schizophrenia has shown deficiencies in autophagy.

Autophagy protects the brain by removing defective proteins, clearing out waste material that accumulates, and protecting against cognitive decline. It keeps neurons healthy and functional and protects against age-related disease by slowing down the aging of brain cells. Autophagy keeps the brain functional and healthy for longer. It is an important process for maintaining much-needed balance in the brain.

Neurodegenerative disorders are often the result of dysfunctional proteins in neurons. Diseases such as Huntington's disease, Alzheimer's, and Parkinson's disease may manifest themselves somewhat differently, but they all share an important similarity. Each disorder is characterized by excessive buildup of proteins inside neurons in the brain. This dysfunction gradually leads to brain cell death and loss of cognitive abilities. Autophagy removes the problematic proteins that are specifically associated with these diseases. This process can significantly reduce your risk of developing dementia or other neurodegenerative disorders. It may also help to treat these conditions after some symptoms have appeared.

Skin Health

Healthy-looking skin can make you look and feel younger, fresher, and more energetic.

When skin cells accumulate damage and toxins, they begin to age. The human body makes new skin cells often, but it generally takes about three months for you to replace all of your skin fully. The process of autophagy expels toxins from the body, which is beneficial for skin health. It helps repair existing cells so that your skin looks and feels healthier. By undergoing autophagy, the skin becomes more resilient and less likely to develop conditions such as eczema, acne, and wrinkles.

This process also helps tighten saggy skin, especially the kind that comes from weight loss. Your body reabsorbs the skin that you no longer need during autophagy, including wrinkles and loose skin.

CHAPTER 7:

Common Mistakes During Intermittent Fasting and How to Avoid Them

Intermittent Fasting is a great process that can bring exemplary health effects. However, any process can only work efficiently if its execution is right and silly mistakes are not done in the execution.

Pay Attention to Macronutrients

The people who are suffering from obesity simply want to get rid of this malice. They are ready to barter anything for it. They dream of a slender figure as the ultimate goal and this is where they become susceptible to make some of the most fatal mistakes.

Intermittent fasting or any form of dieting or calorie-restrictive routine would put certain restrictions on you. Intermittent fasting doesn't put a cap on the amount of food you can eat or its type. However, that doesn't mean you can eat a lot. In most cases, you will have only 7-8 hours in reality to eat anything that you want. Missing that meal may mean that you'll have to go without food till the next meal. Therefore, the amount of food you can eat gets limited.

Other calorie-restrictive routines put an explicit cap on the amount and type of food you can have. You may experience weight loss but that doesn't mean that you are getting healthy.

Your body can only get healthy when it is getting all the macro and micronutrients in the right quantity. It also needs vitamins and minerals. Getting all that while consuming limited calories can be difficult. If you don't pay proper attention here, you will end up with nutrient deficiencies.

You may get a slender frame but you will be battling with more problems than you started with.

Intermittent fasting allows you a proper chance to do so as it doesn't put restrictions on the quantity and types of food items you can have.

The best way to pass this trick with qualifying marks is to have a very balanced meal. Your meals should be high in fat, moderate in protein, and low in carbs.

Before you begin to question the credibility of the suggestion, I would like to clarify some misconceptions:

Fat Is Not Bad

There is a popular misconception that eating fat is bad. Fat is the building block of life. Our body cannot function without fat. Fat, in general, is not bad. Trans fat or the poor-quality fat that we get in processed food is bad. Fat in itself is a form of compact energy. Our body doesn't classify food as fat, protein, or cholesterol. Everything that you eat gets processed and is broken down as calories. This means that fat would also get converted to glucose, and so would happen with carbs. The benefit of eating fat is that you will be able to get more calories in a single meal in comparison to carbs.

Fat is very compact in nature and has almost double the number of calories per gram when compared to carbs. So, if you get 8 calories per gram of carbs, you'll get 16 from fat. Protein is also heavier and has more calories than carbs. This means that if you consume a high–fat low–carb diet, you can get more calories. It also means that even if you have fewer meals in a day, you will not get energy deficient.

Fat should be consumed in greater quantities. You should select high-quality fat. The same goes for protein. You can get protein from animals and cereals and it would help you in muscle building and staying fit. The biggest advantage of having a high-fat, moderate protein, low-carb diet is that it doesn't make you feel hungry very often. Fat and protein content in your meals would help you in transitioning from one meal to the other easily without facing the need to have snacks.

Fat and protein-rich diets also contain a lot of minerals and vitamins. However, the highest part of minerals and vitamins, and fiber should be obtained from carbs. You should consume a lot of leafy green vegetables, salads, whole grain foods. Leafy greens are bulky and but they do not weigh much. They don't add too many calories to your system but they provide most of the vitamins, minerals, phytonutrients, antioxidants, and trace minerals required by your body. You can have leafy green vegetables as much as you want without worrying about calories.

This is a part that you should never undermine in your pursuit to have a slender figure. If you ignore your health, the weight would come back faster than you can lose it. It will also have a very adverse impact on your health.

You must always remember that you need to be healthy to fight weight and it isn't the other way around. The people who lose their weight drastically without a solid base are called sick and not healthy.

You must never forget the macronutrients in your meal as they would become the pillars of your health.

Don't Get Greedy in the Feasting Windows

Food has its own temptation. It looks like the most alluring thing in the world when you have been deprived of it for a long time. This would happen with you too. But it is important that you don't get greedy at such times and lose control. It is very important that you get off your fasting windows in a proper manner.

This can cause several problems and poor digestion is one among them. In the fasting state, the gut gets to stay away from food for extended periods and hence it can get a bit dry. Stuffing it with heavy food can cause problems.

You should also mind the quantity of food that you eat. Our brain takes much longer to understand the leptin signals that you are full. The best way out is to either eat slowly as this would give your brain the time to assess your satiety levels. You can also stop eating when you feel that you are 80% full. Generally, by this time you would have eaten your fill. If you want to test this, you can wait for some time after feeling 80% full and you'd find that you are no longer feeling hungry. It happens as the fat cells are able to properly communicate to the brain that it doesn't need to eat anymore.

Don't Try to Rush the Process

Slow and steady wins the race. This is an adage we all have heard but most of us fail to believe. We want quick results and for that, we are ready to make the jumps. However, this is not how the body works. Your body makes the transition very slowly. It needs the time to adjust to any kind of change positive or negative and the same would happen even in the case of intermittent fasting.

If you want to succeed with the process, you must ensure that you stick to every stage for some time. There would be decades-old habits that would need to change and it can be difficult for your body at times.

Fasting in men and women is completely different. Men have a very rugged system and it doesn't get affected by a bit extended fasting schedule. However, it isn't the case with women. If you try to jerk your system a bit harder, it can affect your health adversely. Your hormonal system may go for a spin and it may take very long for it to normalize. A woman's body reacts very differently to stress signals and hence caution and patience are essential.

Start with the easiest process and give your body the time to adjust to the small breaks. Once it gets used to a certain amount of break, try to extend it a bit slowly. Don't do anything very fast. Always go step by step and you will get your goal easily and without unnecessary difficulties.

Perseverance Is the Key

Impatience is a big problem in people battling with weight. There is no fault of theirs as they are already under great pressure. Most people trying to lose weight have already faced disappointment with other weight loss measures and hence they want to see the results fast to believe them. They are not ready to wait very long to get the results.

This is a point where problems can occur. Intermittent fasting is not any wonder-process. It is a wonderful process but it doesn't work by magic. It tries to correct the problems that may have reached their current state of development in decades at least.

It would take some time for the results to come. You will have to work patiently and not lose hope while the results come. If you quit in between, you wouldn't be able to know if you were making any progress or not. It isn't a process that works overnight. It would require you to take the leap of faith and invest your time and energy into it.

Don't Frame Unrealistic Expectations

We all like to dream big and that is a good thing. However, we must also remain grounded in reality. This will help in accepting the facts and save a lot of disappointments. Many times, we are so engrossed with the imaginary expectations that we fail to recognize the gifts we get. If weight loss is your goal then think of the amount of time you are ready to devote, the lengths to which you can go for it and the medical conditions you are facing. Without considering all these facts, expecting a complete makeover would be absurd. If you have made such expectations, then you will not even be able to enjoy the weight loss you are observing. Your expectations would overshadow the results. It is important that you remain realistic.

Properly Manage Your Fasting Time

It isn't unusual for some people to mismanage their time. Most of us do it in our daily lives. However, poor management of the fasting time can be a cause of great distress for you. It can make your weight loss journey difficult and painful. You cannot remain thinking about food all the while you are in the fasted state. This would create problems for you and your gut would also remain confused.

The best way to manage the fasting time is to keep yourself busy. The last leg of your fasting window should always be planned in such a way that you remain aptly engaged. The idler you are the higher are the chances that you'll only think about food.

Engaging in heavy physical activity is one of the best ways to put off hunger. Hunger in today's age is a highly psychological phenomenon. Our bodies have ample energy stores to run without food for months. It is our mind that is always drawing us towards food. You only need to stall it for a few hours.

Walking, running, laughing, talking to friends, engaging in serious discussions are some of the ways through which we can stall hunger and remain unaffected.

These are some of the common mistakes that we make and which can mar the results we get. Intermittent fasting is a very simple and easy way to lose weight. It doesn't require much of your time and effort. You only need to make up your mind once and bring it into your life. Even if you are following any other weight loss measure, intermittent fasting can still fit into your lifestyle.

CHAPTER 8:

Advantages and Disadvantages of Intermittent Fasting

Female participants in studies across the globe and those reporting their personal results on social media or within fitness communities report many of the same negative effects felt by men throughout the course of adjusting to a new Intermittent Fasting plan. Some of these side effects include:
- Initial hunger pangs and dehydration
- Difficulty concentrating or gaining focus throughout the day
- Headaches, muscle weakness, initial loss in muscle tone

There are some effects that women have experienced and should be watched out for, especially those with a history of trouble or concerns with their menstrual cycles. One such negative effect reported is infertility after long periods of time on an Intermittent Fasting plan. This tends to happen more in women who see a dramatic loss in body fat, especially in the first few weeks (or during the adjustment time).
- In most women, this is nothing to be permanently concerned about as typically periods return to normal and fertility increases in the weeks after stopping an Intermittent Fasting plan, particularly for weight-loss reasons
- Most wellness experts and medical professionals recommend that women who may be pregnant, are pregnant, or are hoping to become pregnant in the near future avoid starting or cease their Intermittent Fasting plan in order to ensure they are in peak condition for childbearing or do not minimize their chances of conceiving

However, for those worried about starting an Intermittent Fasting routine, it is important to point out that even though fasting is still being studied around the world for its long-term benefits and risks on nearly anyone who could ever be interested in trying it (different ages, genders, races, cultural diets, health histories), health and wellness experts all over have written and spoken about its safety, its benefits and its promising progress for men and women alike.

Advantages of Intermittent Fasting

Intermittent fasting has incredible benefits not only to women's bodies and brains but also to men. The following are a few of the benefits linked to intermittent starvation:

Brain health: Since intermittent fasting is better for your body, then it is best for your brain. The reduction of oxidative stress and various worries is advantageous for your brain fitness. Recurrent fasting increases the development of new nerves, which improves the functioning of your brain. It also helps in increasing brain hormone levels known as the Brain-derived neurotrophic factors, which help fight depression and any other brain-related illnesses. Intermittent fasting also helps fight brain damages caused by stroke.

Extending lifespan: Intermittent fasting can help you live longer due to its ability to control metabolism rates, regulating blood sugar levels, and eliminating any dysfunctional cells within your body.

Disadvantages of Intermittent Fasting

Unfortunately, intermittent fasting has cons too, especially for females. Studies show that before trying intermittent fasting, you should always contact your physician. The following are the disadvantages associated with intermittent fasting:

It is not risk-free: Intermittent fasting is not advisable to people who are at higher health risks such as those over sixty-five years. People under medical conditions, high fat needs, the diabetic, the underweight, the underage, pregnant, and those breastfeeding cannot undertake intermittent fasting.

You will be hungry: During intermittent fasting, you might have a grumbling stomach, especially if you have correctly been observing the correct dietary plans. You should avoid looking at, smelling, or even thinking about food while fasting since these triggers the releasing o gastric acids in your stomach, which then makes you hungry. Engage in some other activities but if you wish to fill your water, drink herbal tea or other drinks free from calories. You may note increased food intake in the non-eating days where you are not limited to any calorie intakes. Intermittent fasting triggers binge food consumption. There could also be cases of cravings, especially after increased levels of cortisol hormone.

Dehydration: Lack of eating may make you forget to take water. You might fail to take note of the thirst cues when fasting.

Fatigue: Intermittent fasting makes you feel tired, especially if you are trying it for the first time. Your body tends to run short of energy and disrupts your sleep patterns, and this comes along with a feeling of being tired.

Irritability: Since intermittent fasting helps in mood regulation, it can as well regulate your appetite. It leads to being depressed and upset.

Intermittent fasting long-term consequences are not known: Since no one knows whether after losing weight, you will maintain the same for some years, studies claim that no relevant evidence to support the extent of intermittent fasting. You are therefore always advised to talk to your doctor for sound advice on how you should practice intermittent fasting.

Since you are fasting, it is an obstacle to associating with your friends who are having fun; eating chocolates and drinking wine since you will get tempted to take some. You can indulge in other ways of having fun with your friends. You can pay a visit to the nearest mall, window-shop new clothes or electronics. Avoid grocery stores and any dinner dates. Clear any mouth-watering photos from your gallery.

Avoid getting stressed since stress increases the levels of cortisol, which is responsible for fat storage and muscle breakdown. You can practice yoga, meditating, or having deep breaths. Your body needs enough energy to last you during the fasting period, and so these exercises should be light and not vigorous.

To avoid freaking out, you can always invite your friends to accompany you in doing intermittent fasting. The idea of creating your fasting thread or checking online for any other people doing intermittent fasting can help you master your progress. That is the time that you should focus on mentally cleaning your closet and reflecting on what you are doing.

Avoid 'Victory Binging.' Many people indulge themselves after the fasting period. You should take in a healthy meal and avoid foods that cannot get digested easily. You should take in foods rich in fiber and if you are alcoholic, remember to take care when resuming.

CHAPTER 9:

Pathologies and Cases for Which Intermittent Fasting Is Not Recommended

There are many benefits to intermittent fasting, such as increased metabolism and reduced appetite.

But there are also certain people who should not try this diet because it could be dangerous to their health. These include pregnant women, children, diabetics and people with eating disorders, or those who need to regulate their blood sugar levels.

People with heart problems should also consult a doctor before beginning intermittent fasting because they may be at a higher risk of cardiovascular events like heart attacks and arrhythmias if they go without food for long periods of time.

Intermittent fasting may promote heart health in some people but in others, it could make existing problems worse. According to Martin Berkhan from Leangains.com, there is no evidence that intermittent fasting can cure heart issues, so it is best to check with a doctor before trying it out.

In addition, he says that intermittent fasting can reduce workout performance in athletes, and "many [athletes] have found themselves unable to perform in the gym at their accustomed level". This could be particularly problematic for people with existing eating disorders or who have an unhealthy relationship with food because they might develop an even more negative outlook on food when they start fasting and lose control of their eating habits altogether.

Intermittent fasting could also be dangerous for pregnant women because it can put them at a higher risk of complications during childbirth. Pregnant women are already at risk of losing their baby or suffering from other complications like pre-eclampsia, which is why they must eat properly and stay hydrated when they're expecting.

But when they fast, this could put their nutrition levels too low and increase their chances of this occurring. Berkhan says that "in studies in which subjects are calorie-restricted, miscarriages are frequent as the body tries to protect the fetus in any way possible."

Children also cannot benefit from intermittent fasting because they still need proper nutrition, especially when their bodies are developing at such a rapid rate. As Berkhan says, "they are still growing and developing and need the nutrition to build their bodies."

Eating disorders like anorexia nervosa can also cause problems when people try intermittent fasting because it could make them lose control of their eating habits even more and trigger binge-eating episodes. And those with bulimia nervosa might end up causing potentially fatal damage to their digestive system by consuming large amounts of calories while fasting.

People with type 1 diabetes should also go through a proper consultation before starting intermittent fasting because it could affect how much insulin they require throughout the day. As Berkhan says, test subjects who fasted lost significant amounts of insulin sensitivity, which could cause them to get very sick if they don't adjust their intake of the hormone properly.

According to Charles Poliquin, a strength coach and author of Strength Training: 3rd Edition, people with eating disorders like anorexia nervosa might start struggling even more when they try intermittent fasting. This is because it could make them get anxious about food and jeopardize their recovery by making their minds more preoccupied with the process of eating than with getting better.

So as these people try to recover from their eating disorders, it is best that they refrain from fasting or at least do so under supervision by a professional.

Berkhan says that "insulin sensitivity is decreased during fasting," so those who already have an impaired ability to produce insulin might end up getting ill if they try intermittent fasting without consulting a doctor first.

In addition, people with eating disorders or those who have problems regulating their blood sugar levels should not try intermittent fasting because it could make these conditions worse and trigger binges or even cause them to relapse. This could be very dangerous for people with diabetes because severe cases of hypoglycemia can cause a coma or even death.

As Berkhan says, "intermittent fasting is not recommended for anyone with an eating disorder or altered hunger regulation as it can cause severe binging episodes and other unhealthy behaviors."

Berkhan also warns against fasting to greater degrees than is recommended because it could be potentially fatal. He says that "if you are already leaner than desired, then don't fast longer than 24 hours." According to him, people who fast for longer periods of time are in danger of developing symptoms like hypoglycemia and ketosis.

He also states that "if you have been doing 24/48 hour fasts for a month or more and have yet to see any fat loss results, then something else is wrong." Fasting for a long time may make weight loss more difficult because the body will get used to storing energy without food.

CHAPTER 10:

What Side Effects Intermittent Fasting Might Have

Some people that swear by this practice might not be willing to admit that there are unpleasant side effects of fasting intermittently. But that might be myopic and withholding vital information.

It's essential to means that the overall downsides of intermittent fasting are common to all or any women no matter age. While women of child-bearing age may need effects on their reproductive hormones, post-menopausal women or older women might not get to worry about reproduction. However, they experience frequent changes in their moods, difficulty in sleeping, and occasional headaches.

After a comprehensive review of several scientific studies on women's health, fasting, and aging, researchers weren't ready to find any significant adverse effects of intermittent fasting and point to a scarcity of research on the subject (Journal of Mid-Life Health, 2016). These sorts of scientific reviews are beneficial for getting unbiased information that provides you a broader picture of several results from different related studies performed over a few years. Comprehensive reviews hamper prejudices often related to smaller researchers that will are sponsored by interest groups. Overall, scientific studies show encouraging leads to different aspects of women's health, including psychological state, physical fitness, and weight loss. That's not to say there are not any adverse side effects of intermittent fasting. It only means the adverse side effects of intermittent fasting are common to women of all ages – both pre and post-menopausal women and depend mainly on the individual woman.

With that being said, not everyone who practices intermittent fasting will have a negative side effect. These differ from person to person. The important thing is being conscious of these adverse side effects and learning the way to handle them if they occur. Also, remember that the majority of the off-putting impacts of intermittent fast don't last beyond the primary few days. Every week or two, your body would have adjusted to your new eating schedule, and any adverse effects will gradually subside until things feel back to normal. So, it's crucial to permit your body a while to regulate rather than trying intermittent fasting for one or two days and throwing in the towel.

Here is the way to affect a number of the common negative side effects you'll likely encounter as you begin your new eating habits.

Hunger

One of the primary not-so-fun and most blatant results of fasting is hunger. This side effect is difficult because going without food longer than your body is conditioned to will end in an uncomfortable desire for love or money to eat. All of your life, you've got programmed your body to expect food at certain times throughout the day. It might be weird if you suddenly change your eating pattern, and your body accepts the change without putting up a minimum of a touch resistance. If your body doesn't get food at the time it usually does, a hormone called ghrelin –

the hunger hormone – will start acting up to remind you that you simply should supply your body with food. This "acting up" or reminder to erode your usual time will continue until your brain convinces ghrelin to accept your new eating schedule simply. But until then, you'll likely feel intense hunger but don't worry; it'll pass. You'll get to tap into your reserve of mental strength to remain committed to your course.

To effectively handle hunger pangs, drink more water, or any qualifying beverage on intermittent fasting. Doing so will help to suppress hunger pangs. Very often, the sensation of hunger isn't necessarily a sign that you simply are hungry; it'd be a small dip in your blood glucose level – something that water or other non-calorie liquids can look out of.

To help delay hunger on your fasting days or in the fasting window (depending on the sort of fasting regimen you select to follow), make sure that you include adequate amounts of healthy fats, carbs, and proteins in your meals before commencing your fast. Also, when fasting, try to take your mind off food. Combining low-impact exercises with fasting can assist in giving you the boost you would like to travel through your day without feeling too uncomfortable. Getting enough sleep also will help you throughout the day; there's nothing that will upset your day entirely lack of sleep in the dark and having to fast. That's an open invitation for fatigue and hunger!

Frequent Urination

As with hunger, it's also expected to experience a rise in the number of times you urinate. There is no mystery here as intermittent fasting takes that you simply increase your intake of water and other liquids to remain hydrated. This effect may successively increase the frequency of urination. Keep drinking your water, and don't avoid bathroom visits. Holding it for too long can weaken your bladder muscles, and trying not to drink water will soon cause you to be dehydrated and supply subsequent side effects – both bad!

Headaches

Intermittent fasting can make your blood glucose take a nosedive. This fact introduces stress on your body, your brain will release stress hormones, and you'll likely experience a point of headache. Dehydration can cause headaches in intermittent fasting as your body tells you it lacks adequate water.

To reduce the occurrence of headaches, attempt to minimize stress on your body. It's okay to exercise in fasting, but excessive exercise can trigger an excessive amount of stress. Also, attempt to keep your body hydrated in the least times by drinking enough water. But don't chug water in a rush and don't drink water excessively. An excessive amount of water may result in an imbalance in your mineral and body water ratio.

Cravings

It is normal to experience quite usual cravings for food in your fasting window. This fact is often a biological and psychological response to the sensation of deprivation that's often related to going without food. And since your body is all bent to get glucose, you would possibly notice that you simply crave more sugar or carbohydrates. These cravings don't mean that you simply are less committed to your goals. Instead, cravings happen to remind you that you simply are human. Even ardent practitioners of intermittent fasting experience cravings from time to time.

When you start looking for something, remind yourself of your goal and distract yourself from food-related topics. Keep your mind engrossed with other non-food-related activities like hobbies, talking and enter nature, or getting to sleep for a short time. In your eating window, you'll treat yourself to a healthy bite of what you crave to attenuate the intensity of the craving or longing. Remind yourself in your fasting window that you simply will soon eat what you long for, so there's no need to dwell thereon or giving it an excessive amount of thought when it's not yet time to eat. Remind your body that you simply are not any longer an adolescent or a young adult. You've got had many experiences in curbing your cravings, and this case isn't an exception.

Heartburn, Bloating, and Constipation

Occasionally, heartburn can occur when your stomach produces acids for digestion of your food, but there's no food present in the stomach to be digested. Bloating and constipation usually go hand in hand and may also occur in some cases. Together, these two can cause you to feel very uncomfortable.

Drinking adequate amounts of water can reduce the danger of heartburn, bloating, and constipation. Heartburns also can be minimized by lowering spicy foods in your eating window. If you experience heartburn in intermittent fasting, here's something you'll try before getting to sleep. Prop yourself up once you lie to sleep. But don't use pillows to prop yourself as it will put more pressure on your stomach and increase the discomfort. Use a specially designed wedge or use a 6-inch block or something almost like elevate your head as you lie. Doing this may make gravity minimize the backward flow of your stomach contents into your gullet. Propping yourself in this manner should bring you relief from heartburn. However, if heartburn, bloating, and constipation persist, consult your doctor immediately.

Binging

Eating an excessive amount as soon because the fasting window is over is typically related to first-timers to fasting. The extreme hunger of fasting can drive you to dine in a rush when breaking, and you'll find yourself overeating. In some cases, binging is often a result of an easy misunderstanding of the fundamentals of intermittent fasting. They assume that they will eat the maximum amount they need in the eating window since the no-eating window will look out for calories. This misunderstanding can deprive you of gaining any significant benefits that accompany fasting intermittently, especially if you're looking to shed some weight. Binging or overeating in your eating window will reverse all the diligence you set in in the fast.

To avoid binging, make sure that the dimensions and meals are planned well before the eating window. Don't start fasting without knowing what portion you're getting to consume at the top. Waiting until you'll eat to make a decision about what to eat and the way much to eat can cause overeating because your food choices are going to be primarily influenced by how hungry you are feeling.

Low Energy

Feeling exhausted may be a standard part of fasting. Until your body gets won't to sourcing its fuel from fat storage, you're likely to experience some decline in your energy levels. Usually, they revisit up in a few days.

To help stay energized, tailor your activities to remain low-key, a minimum of initially. There's no got to push yourself to prove that you simply are a robust woman. Deciding to practice intermittent fasting is enough proof that you simply are mentally, emotionally, and physically healthy.

Since you're not in competition with anyone, it's in your best interest to conserve energy the maximum amount possible. Get a massage, spend time relaxing in bed, or sleeping in if you've got to. These little activities can go an extended way to keep you energized.

Feeling Cold

Some people experience an additional feeling of cold in fasting. If you experience this, there's no cause for alarm. It'd be a result of the drop in your blood glucose level. Usually, blood flow to your internal fat storage is increased in fasting. This increase results in fat moved to parts of the body where it needs to be used as energy. This effect will make other parts of your body that have less fat storage experience cold. So, if you feel cold in your fingers or toes, it's your body doing its fat burning process for your good.

To help reduce the cold, place on layers, stay in warm areas, drink hot coffee or tea (with no calories), or take a hot shower. It's important to keep in mind that feeling cold is simply a result of intermittent fasting and doesn't mean you're ill. So, avoid the urge to self-medicate. If the cold feeling persists even in your non-fasting days or in your eating window, consult your doctor.

CHAPTER 11:

How Intermittent Fasting Will Help People Over 50

How Intermittent Fasting Will Affect Women Over 50 Differently

Some of the diseases or health-related issues that are more likely to affect women over the age of 50 include joint pain, arthritis, lower metabolism (which can lead to weight gain), reduced muscle mass, sleep disturbances, increased levels of belly fat, osteoporosis and other common but weight and age-related diseases such as heart disease or diabetes. By practicing intermittent fasting and losing weight; as a result, you will reduce your risk of developing several of these diseases. By inducing autophagy, you are reducing your risk of those diseases that are not as closely related to weight, such as cancer and heart attacks.

Joint Health

In women over 50, there is much more risk of developing joint issues such as knee pain, wrist, elbow, or shoulder pain. This is due to an increase in age and more risk of arthritis or low back and other joint pain due to age and overuse. In studies where women over 50 practiced intermittent fasting for a period of time, they were found to have decreased levels of joint pain, arthritic symptoms, and low back pain.

How Women Over 50 Can Benefit from Intermittent Fasting

As you have seen evidenced throughout this book, intermittent fasting is extremely beneficial for women over 50, and most of the research done around this type of diet regime points to positive effects. It is quite difficult to find research that doesn't support intermittent fasting for women over 50 as an effective tool for weight loss, improved health, and better overall mental health. As long as intermittent fasting is followed in a safe manner, the results can be extremely positive!

Things for Women Over 50 to Keep in Mind

Supplementing may be very beneficial and even necessary when fasting to maintain and improve health. If you are fasting, it may be difficult to obtain sufficient amounts of essential nutrients and minerals, such as Omega-3 or iron. For this reason, supplementing them may benefit you in terms of keeping you feeling healthy and energetic, as well as keeping your brain functioning to its full potential. You can take specific nutrients on their own in pill form or you can opt for a multivitamin that will include all of the most essential vitamins and minerals for overall good health. These vitamins and minerals may differ from those that we looked at in the previous chapter, as those included the vitamins and minerals that are known to induce autophagy. The vitamins included in a multivitamin will be those that are known to promote good overall health and those that are usually obtained through a balanced, whole food diet.

Nutrients You Need and How to Get Them

For women over 50, it is important to make sure that you get all the nutrients your body needs, especially if you are trying to lose weight or following treatments that include fasting. To ensure that during your fasting periods, you are as healthy as possible, supplementation is something that could be considered, to ensure that you are feeding your body the nutrients it needs. Below, we will look at some whole food sources as well as some supplements that you may wish to consider.

Omega 3 Fatty Acids

These are something that is essential since they cannot be made in our bodies. Omega-3 Fatty Acids are substances that are necessary to get from your diet as the body cannot make them on its own. These fatty acids are a certain type in a list of other fatty acids, but this type (Omega-3) is the most essential and the most beneficial for our brains and bodies in general. They have numerous effects on the brain including reducing inflammation (which reduces the risk of Alzheimer's) and maintaining and improving mood and cognitive function, including memory. Omega-3's has these greatly beneficial effects because of the way that they act in the brain, which is what makes them so essential to our diets. Omega-3 Fatty Acids increase the production of new nerve cells in the brain by acting specifically on the nerve stem cells within the brain, causing new and healthy nerve cells to be generated.

Omega-3 fatty acids can be found in fish like salmon, sardines, black cod, and herring. It can also be taken as a pill-form supplement for those who do not eat fish or cannot eat enough of it. It can also be taken in the form of a fish oil supplement like krill oil.

Omega-3's is by far the most important nutrient that you need to ensure you are ingesting because of the numerous benefits that come from it, both in the brain and in the rest of the body. While supplements are often the last step when it comes to trying to include something in your diet, for Omega-3's the benefits are too great to potentially miss by trying to receive all of it from your diet.

Sulforaphane

Brussels Sprouts, Cabbage, Kale, Broccoli Sprouts have in common? All of these green vegetables have one thing in common- they all contain Sulforaphane. Sulforaphane is a plant chemical that is found naturally in these vegetables. This is an antioxidant that acts in a similar way to turmeric and thus has similar benefits. Sulforaphane like turmeric induces autophagy in the brain which helps to reduce the risk of Alzheimer's, Parkinson's and dementia which are all neurodegenerative diseases. Neurodegenerative means that the cells in the brain called nerves are damaged and broken down, which leads to cognitive declines like Alzheimer's or physical decline as in Parkinson's. These vegetables can help to treat these diseases by slowing their progression, as they are all diseases that come about over time. There is no cure yet, but the treatment at this stage involves delaying the progression of these diseases.

Sulforaphane can be found in the aforementioned vegetables, but the strongest source is broccoli sprouts. It can also be taken concentrated in a supplement form.

Calcium

Calcium is beneficial for the healthy circulation of blood, and for maintaining strong bones and teeth. Calcium can come from dairy products like milk, yogurt, and cheese. It can also be found in leafy greens like kale and broccoli and sardines.

Magnesium

Magnesium is beneficial for your diet, as it also helps you to maintain strong bones and teeth. Magnesium and Calcium are most effective when ingested together, as Magnesium helps in the absorption of calcium. It also helps to reduce migraines and is great for calmness and relieving anxiety. Magnesium can be found in leafy green vegetables like kale and spinach, as well as fruits like bananas and raspberries, legumes like beans and chickpeas, vegetables like peas, cabbage, green beans, asparagus and Brussels sprouts, and fish like tuna and salmon.

Exogenous Ketones

When tested on animal models, even when they were ingested on a normal carbohydrate intake diet, these exogenous ketones proved to be beneficial in terms of helping the models with problems like seizures, being anti-cancer, anti-inflammation, and anti-anxiety, which are the diseases that we normally see to be assisted by ketosis (which is the state the body enters when it is using fat as a source of fuel instead of carbohydrates), just like we saw in the first few chapters of this book.

Electrolytes

When you first begin following an intermittent fasting regime, having Electrolyte depletion is quite common. This is because of water weight loss through fat and a lower carbohydrate intake, which is often common, as we have discussed. Taking electrolyte supplements can help to avoid a deficiency in common electrolytes, like magnesium, potassium and sodium. This is also why you should ensure you are getting enough dietary sodium, as this is an electrolyte that you need. Along with this, though, you will need to ensure you are drinking enough water to avoid dehydration.

Iron

This one is a little tricky, but it is worth noting. Iron should be obtained in the right amounts in your diet through whole foods. Iron cannot be supplemented without being referred by a doctor first, as it is something that they would like you to first try to get from your food. If this is becoming a problem, they can give you supplements to take.

Vitamin D

Vitamin D is found in some foods that have been fortified with it, but in a natural sense, it can be found in only a few foods. These include cheese, fatty fish like salmon and tuna as well as egg yolks. Another source is mushrooms that have been exposed to UV rays, so the organic ones are likely of this sort. Vitamin D can be absorbed naturally through sun exposure, so if you live in a sunny place, make sure you get us for some walks or some timer with the sun on your skin. If you live in a colder or gloomier place, consider purchasing a lamp that mimics the sun and provides you with vitamin D in your house. On a sunny day, even if it is cold going outside and getting sun on your face will give you vitamin D.

This one is something that everyone should be conscious of, but it is especially necessary to examine if you are following a specific diet.

Bioactive Compounds

Bioactive compounds are compounds found within foods that act in the body in beneficial ways. The bioactive compounds found within berries, such as Acai Berries, Strawberries, and Blueberries are very beneficial for your health. The bioactive compounds in these specific types of berries work in the brain to induce autophagy and reduce inflammation. This leads to the protection of brain cells in this case from oxidative stress. Oxidative stress is something that can happen within the brain when there is an imbalance of oxygen, which can cause reduced cognitive functioning. These berries and their induction of autophagy helps to reduce this by keeping the balance of oxygen at a healthy level.

CHAPTER 12:

What Happens and What Are the Changes in the Human Body with Menopause

Menopause is one of the most complicated phases in a woman's life. The time when our bodies begin to change and important natural transitions occur that are too often negatively affected, while it is important to learn how to change our eating habits and eating patterns appropriately. In fact, it often happens that a woman is not ready for this new condition and experiences it with a feeling of defeat as an inevitable sign of time travel, and this feeling of prostration turns out to be too invasive and involves many aspects of one's stomach.

It is therefore important to remain calm as soon as there are messages about the first signs of change in our human body, to ward off the onset of menopause for the right purpose, and to minimize the negative effects of suffering, especially in the early days. Even during this difficult transition, targeted nutrition can be very beneficial.

What Happens to the Body of a Menopausal Woman?

It must be said that a balanced diet has been carried out in life and there are no major weight fluctuations, this will no doubt be a factor that supports women who are going through menopause, but that it is not a sufficient condition to present with classic symptoms that are felt, which can be classified according to the period experienced. In fact, we can distinguish between the pre-menopausal phase, which lasts around 45 to 50 years, and is physiologically compatible with a drastic reduction in the production of the hormone estrogen (responsible for the menstrual cycle, which actually starts irregularly). This period is accompanied by a series of complex and highly subjective endocrine changes. Compare effectively: headache, depression, anxiety and sleep disorders.

When someone enters actual menopause, estrogen hormone production decreases even more dramatically, the range of the symptoms widens, leading to large amounts of the hormone, for example, to a certain class called catecholamine adrenaline. The result of these changes is a dangerous heat wave, increased sweating, and the presence of tachycardia, which can be more or less severe.

However, the changes also affect the female genital organs, with the volume of the breasts, uterus and ovaries decreasing. The mucous membranes become less active and vaginal dryness increases. There may also be changes in bone balance, with decreased calcium intake and increased mobilization at the expense of the skeletal system. Because of this, there is a lack of continuous bone formation, and conversely, erosion begins, which is a predisposition for osteoporosis.

Although menopause causes major changes that greatly change a woman's body and soul, metabolism is one of the worst. In fact, during menopause, the absorption and accumulation of sugars and triglycerides changes and it is easy to increase some clinical values such as cholesterol and triglycerides, which lead to high blood pressure or arteriosclerosis. In addition, many women often complain of disturbing circulatory disorders and local edema, especially in the stomach. It also makes weight gain easier, even though you haven't changed your eating habits.

The Ideal Diet for Menopause

In cases where disorders related to the arrival of menopause become difficult to manage, drug or natural therapy under medical supervision may be necessary. The contribution given by a correct diet at this time can be considerable, in fact, given the profound variables that come into play, it is necessary to modify our food routine, both in order not to be surprised by all these changes, and to adapt in the most natural way possible.

The problem of fat accumulation in the abdominal area is always caused by the drop in estrogen. In fact, they are also responsible for the classic hourglass shape of most women, which consists of depositing fat mainly on the hips, which begins to fail with menopause. As a result, we go from a gynoid condition to an android one, with an adipose increase localized on the belly. In addition, the metabolic rate of disposal is reduced, this means that even if you do not change your diet and eat the same quantities of food as you always have, you could experience weight gain, which will be more marked in the presence of bad habits or irregular diet.

The digestion is also slower and intestinal function becomes more complicated. This further contributes to swelling as well as the occurrence of intolerance and digestive disorders which have never been disturbed before. Therefore, the beginning will be more problematic and difficult to manage during this period. The distribution of nutrients must be different: reducing the amount of low carbohydrate, which is always preferred not to be purified, helps avoid the peak of insulin and at the same time maintains stable blood sugar.

Furthermore, it will be necessary to slightly increase the quantity of both animal and vegetable proteins; choose good fats, preferring seeds and extra virgin olive oil, and severely limit saturated fatty acids (those of animal origin such as lard, lard, etc.). All this to try to increase the proportion of antioxidants taken, which will help to counteract the effect of free radicals, whose concentration begins to increase during this period. It will be necessary to prefer foods rich in phytoestrogens, which will help to control the states of stress to which the body is subjected and which will favor, at least in part, the overall estrogenic balance.

These molecules are divided into three main groups and the foods that contain them should never be missing on our tables: isoflavones, present mainly in legumes such as soy and red clover; lignans, of which flax seeds and oily seeds, in general, are particularly rich; coumestans, found in sunflower seeds, beans and sprouts. A calcium supplementation will be necessary through cheeses such as parmesan; dairy products such as yogurt, egg yolk, some vegetables such as rocket, Brussels sprouts, broccoli, spinach, asparagus; legumes; dried fruit such as nuts, almonds or dried grapes.

Excellent additional habits that will help to regain well-being may be: limiting sweets to sporadic occasions, thus drastically reducing sugars (for example by giving up sugar in coffee and getting used to drinking it bitterly); learn how to dose alcohol a lot (avoiding spirits, liqueurs, and aperitif drinks) and choose only one glass of good wine when you are in company, this because it tends to increase visceral fat which is precisely what is going to settle at the level abdominal. Clearly, even by eating lots of fruit, it is difficult to reach a high carbohydrate quota as in a traditional diet. However, a dietary plan to follow can be useful to have a more precise indication on how to distribute the foods. Obviously, one's diet must be structured in a personal way, based on specific metabolic needs and one's lifestyle.

CHAPTER 13:

How Intermittent Fasting Can Help and Menopause Women

How to Use Intermittent Fasting in Your Menopause Stage?

Some claims suggest that intermittent fasting needs to be modified during menopause, which is true to a certain degree and easily achieved with easier fasting protocols. In general, most women, even during menopause have no problem with intermittent fasting, and the problems start to occur only if you attempt fasts that are longer than 48hours.

Nonetheless, you should know the claims and studies done on women regarding intermittent fasting. There was one study suggesting that blood sugar worsened in women after three weeks of intermittent fasting. Moreover, many sources are claiming that irreversible and damaging changes in women's menstrual cycle will occur with an intermittent fasting schedule which we have discussed in previous chapters.

Hence, people believe that women should not do intermittent fasting, which we disagree with. If done tastefully, intermittent fasting has resulted in excellent health and weight loss benefits for women. If you have reached age fifty, then you should congratulate yourself. You have been through school, teen years, relationships, children, and, most importantly, the changing of your body. You might be looking at your body and asking it exactly what happened during the last few years. Some things you have not been able to control, like hereditary medical issues and the stress that time puts on our bodies. Accidents and illnesses are also beyond our control. But you can begin now to understand the changes in your body and make plans to reduce or eliminate as many of the negative changes as you possibly can.

The first thing that will probably happen to you as you near 50 years of age, is the onset of menopause. The most notable thing about menopause is that your monthly periods will stop – forever! Menopause is the biggest single change that your body will ever experience besides puberty. Menopause can lead to belly fat, weight gain, and osteoporosis. It is a natural occurrence in the life of every woman, caused by the body making less of the hormone's estrogen and progesterone.

Estrogens (there are more than one) is the name for the group of sex-related hormones that make women be women. They cause and promote the initial development and further maintenance of female characteristics in the human body. Estrogens are what gave you breasts, hair in the right places, the ability to reproduce, and your monthly cycle. Estrogen is the hormone that does all of the long-term work in maintaining femininity. Progesterone has one purpose in the woman's body: to implant the egg in the uterus and keep her pregnant until it is time to deliver the baby.

In women, estrogen is crucial to becoming and remaining womanly. In the ovaries, it stimulates the growth of eggs for reproduction. It causes the vagina to grow to proper adult size. Estrogen promotes the healthy growth of the fallopian tubes and the uterus. And it causes your breasts to grow and to fill with milk when a baby arrives. Estrogen is also responsible for making women store some excess fat around their thighs and hips. This weight storage is nature's way of ensuring that the baby will have nutrition during times of famine.

One of the forms of estrogen dramatically decreases in production after menopause, and this form helps women regulate the rate of their metabolism and how fast they gain weight. After menopause, women tend to gain more weight in the middle area of their body, and in the abdomen. This fat collects around the organs and is known as visceral fat. Besides being unattractive, visceral fat is also dangerous because it has been linked to some cancers, heart disease, stroke, and diabetes.

But a lack of estrogen is not the only reason women tend to gain weight after age fifty. Besides a lack of estrogen, the biggest single reason women over fifty gain weight are lifestyle changes. They are no longer running children to activities; so many women move less after fifty. And sometimes they move less because their joints have begun to ache. Stiffness begins to set in, especially in the morning when rolling out of bed suddenly becomes a chore. Many continue to cook large meals and have difficulty scaling back to cooking for just one or two people, and someone needs to eat that food. And some women still feel that life ends when the children leave, so they might as well just indulge a little.

But all of this indulging and relaxing leads to loss of muscle strength, loss of flexibility, and increased belly fat, which in turn leads to even more problems. It also leads to an increased risk for osteoporosis. The lack of estrogen is the leading cause of osteoporosis, which translates literally to porous bone. The bones in the body, particularly the long bones of the arms and the legs, become more porous as the quality and density of the bone are reduced. Bones will continue to regrow and refresh themselves all of your life, but in osteoporosis, the bone is deteriorating faster than new growth can occur.

Estrogen helps to decrease overall cholesterol levels in women, which is why younger women sometimes remain healthy even when they don't take the time to eat healthy meals. All of these changes become more prevalent after fifty and the arrival of menopause because suddenly the estrogen levels drop dramatically. This increase in cholesterol in the body can lead to strokes and heart attacks. Cholesterol is a substance that occurs naturally in your body and is made by the liver. Cholesterol in your body also comes from the foods that you eat. The two kinds that your doctor will measure with a blood test are high-density lipoprotein (HDL) and low-density lipoprotein (LDL). The two numbers together make up your total cholesterol number. Estrogen promotes HDL and depresses LDL, so a lack of estrogen will allow for a higher LDL number.

HDL is the type of cholesterol known as the good type because it removes excess amounts of cholesterol from your arteries and then carries it to the liver to be metabolized and removed from the body during waste removal. LDL is the bad form of cholesterol because it likes to sit in your arteries and form deposits known as plaque. It is possible to have a high total cholesterol number and still be considered healthy if the number is high because HDL is high, and the LDL is low. This means that your body is doing the right thing, and the good cholesterol is eliminating the bad cholesterol.

When LDL clumps in the arteries and forms plaques, it causes hardening of the arteries. Blood will not flow very well through stiff arteries. Your heart will need to work harder to push the blood through your body. And if you have gained a significant amount of weight, your body has created new arteries to supply blood flow to this increased part of you. This will also make the heart work harder than it needs to. And if plaque builds up in the arteries that are connected to the heart, those arteries can become clogged, which results in coronary artery disease. This can cause a heart attack if a piece of plaque breaks loose and cuts off the steady flow of blood to the muscles of the heart. If this happens in the arteries that lead to the brain, it can cause a stroke.

Too much cholesterol has also been found in the brains of people who had Alzheimer's disease. And an excessive amount of cholesterol can cause gallstones, which women are naturally at a higher risk of anyway.

You may have noticed that you seem to be losing control of your bladder function, or that laughing or sneezing makes you leak. This is also a normal effect of aging because the muscles are not as strong as they used to be. Also, the excess weight pressing down on the bladder does not help the situation.

While it is impossible to stop the process of aging, there are things every woman can do to slow the process and help her body remain healthy far into the future. One of the most important ways women can do this is to maintain a healthy weight, which is what makes the keto diet so important for all women and especially for those over age fifty.

CHAPTER 14:

Types of Intermittent Fasting

Intermittent fasting isn't a diet, yet rather a dieting pattern. In less troublesome terms: it's creating a conscious decision to skirt certain meals deliberately.

By fasting and thereafter eating up deliberately, intermittent fasting, all things considered, infers that you exhaust your calories during a significant window of the day, and choose not to eat sustenance for a greater window of time.

5:2 and 4:3 Method

Intermittent fasting is an eating method that incorporates customary fasting.

The 5:2 diet, for the most part, called the 4:3 diet method, generally called The Fast Diet, is, starting at now, the most renowned intermittent fasting diet.

It's known as the 5:2 diet for five days of the week are run-of-the-mill eating days, while the other two limit calories to 500–600 consistently.

Since there are no requirements about which sustenances to eat yet, rather when you should eat them, this diet is, even more, a lifestyle.

Various people see thusly eating as more straightforward to hold fast to than a traditional calorie-restricted diet.

The most effective method to do the 5:2 Diet

The 5:2 diet is, in all actuality, simple to explain. For five days of the week, you usually eat and don't have to consider restricting calories.

By then, on the other two days, you decline your calorie admission to a fourth of your everyday needs. This is around 500 calories every day for women and 650 for men.

You can pick whichever two days of the week you like, as long as there is at any rate one non-fasting day in them.

One standard method for masterminding the week is to fast on Mondays and Thursdays, with a couple of little meals, by then, normally eat for the rest of the week.

Accentuate that eating "ordinarily" doesn't mean you can eat anything. In the event that you gorge on lousy sustenance, by then, you in all probability won't lose any weight anymore, and you may even add more weight.

You should eat a comparable proportion of sustenance just as you hadn't been fasting using any and all means.

Note: The 5:2 diet incorporates routinely eating for five days out of every week by then binding your calorie admission to 500–600 calories on the other two days.

Therapeutic points of interest of 5:2 Intermittent Fasting

There are very few assessments on the 5:2 diet unequivocally.

There is a lot of focuses on intermittent fasting when all is said in done, which shows stunning restorative preferences.

One noteworthy bit of leeway is that intermittent fasting is apparently easier to seek after than interminable calorie control on any occasion for specific people.

Similarly, various assessments have demonstrated that different sorts of intermittent fasting may inside and out diminishing insulin levels.

The 5:2 diet caused weight loss like ordinary calorie restriction. Likewise, the diet was amazingly ground-breaking at decreasing insulin levels and improving insulin affectability.

A couple of studies have researched the prosperity effects of changed substitute day fasting, which is, in a general sense, equivalent to the 5:2 diet (finally, it's a 4:3 diet).

The 4:3 diet may help decline insulin restriction, asthma, intermittent sensitivities, heart arrhythmias, menopausal hot flashes, and anything is possible from that point.

One randomized controlled assessment in both runs of the mill weight and overweight individuals indicated critical upgrades in the get-together doing 4:3 fasting, appeared differently in relation to the control bundle that ate conventionally.

Following 12 weeks, the fasting gathering had:
- Decreased body weight by in excess of 12 pounds (5 kg).
- Reduced fat mass by 7.8 pounds (3.5 kg), with no change in mass.
- Reduced blood levels of triglycerides by 20%.
- Increased LDL atom size, which is something to be appreciative of.
- Reduced degrees of CRP, a huge marker of irritation.
- Reduced degrees of leptin by up to 40%.

The 5:2 diet may have a couple of great therapeutic points of interest, including weight loss, decreased insulin resistance, and lessened irritation. It may moreover improve blood lipids.

The 5:2 Diet for Weight Loss

If you need to get slenderer, the 5:2 diet can be very convincing when done right.

Despite the fact that the 5:2 eating pattern urges you to consume fewer calories.

Consequently, it is critical not to compensate for the fasting days by eating considerably more on no fasting days.

The intermittent fasting plan doesn't include more weight loss than ordinary calorie restriction if all-out calories are composed.

Fasting methods like the 5:2 diet have indicated a huge amount of assurance in weight loss contemplates:
- A late review found that balanced substitute day fasting incited weight loss of 3–8% all through 3–24 weeks.
- In a comparable report, individuals lost 4–7% of their midriff circuit, suggesting that they lost a great arrangement of destructive belly fat.

Intermittent fasting causes a ton of tinier decline in mass when diverged from weight loss with standard calorie restriction. Intermittent fasting is considerably progressively fruitful when gotten together with turn out, for instance, steadiness or quality planning.

20/4

Dissimilar to the Warrior Diet quickly depicted over, the 20:4 Intermittent Fasting protocol utilized by the low-carb network today alternates a protracted fasting period with a customary ketogenic diet.

The long quick enables insulin to remain low for an all-encompassing period.

The "20" in the 20:4 recipe implies you go 20 hours without eating anything, including ketogenic nourishments.

Everything you can have is no-calorie fluids.

The 20 hours quick is known as the fasting window.

The "4" in the 20:4 equation implies you eat an ordinary keto diet during the four sequential hours that you're not fasting.

The 4 hours eating period is known as the meal eating window.

You need not restrain you're eating to simply night times. You can suit your 20 hours of fasting and 4-hour eating window to accommodate your inclinations, hunger level, and what's happening in your life.

Food to Eat During 20:4 Intermittent Fasting

There has been lots of research on fasting done throughout the years. However, a large portion of the work has been done on creatures, and specifically — mice.

Sadly, look into discoveries that apply to mice don't constantly associate with people, so the vast majority of the data that is accessible on what to eat and drink for an effective fasting system is exceptionally abstract.

Standard rules for a 20:4 quick are to not eat or drink anything during the fasting hours that contain calories.

A few dieters carefully adhere to this standard, while others don't.

Out of the entirety of the intermittent fasting choices, a 20:4 arrangement is probably the strictest program to go with, so not every person has the ability to stay with that 4-hour window, particularly the individuals who are accustomed to getting a charge out of a little twofold cream and sugar substitute in their espresso toward the beginning of the day.

Numerous dieters will drink Bullet-Proof Coffee in the first part of the day and afterward eat during their 4-hour window around evening time.

Others are hungrier during the day and think that it's simpler to plan their eating during breakfast or lunch and afterward forego eating around evening time.

Regardless of which window outline you use, or what number of meals you eat all through those 4 hours, the agreement on nourishment is to stay with a low-carb diet.

Some even go zero carbs.

A low-carb diet is characterized as under 30 carbs a day; with most dieters fitting, they are a couple of meals to a limit of 20 carbs or less.

Substituting Fasting

Interchange Day Intermittent Fasting

Interchange day intermittent fasting is basically fasting each other day for a 24-hour period. For instance, you would usually eat on Monday, speedy Tuesday, eat Wednesday, prompt Thursday, eat Friday, snappy Saturday, and so forth.

This use of intermittent fasting is the most standard structure used in inquire about inspects, yet from what I have seen, it isn't outstandingly pervasive actually. I've never endeavored exchange day fasting myself, and I don't plan to do it in that capacity.

In my eyes, it's somewhat excessive, and a considerable part of the negative effects found in specific women while fasting will, as a rule, be related to this sort of fasting.

Additionally, it looks good since you're not eating a small amount of the time, which isn't judicious, especially for women for whom carbs and caloric confirmation are huge for hormones and wealth.

If this is the essential method you endeavor as you understand how to do intermittent fasting, my fear is that it will be unreasonably hard for you, and you'll give up everything together.

Genuinely, it's just not reasonable for by far most with the exception of on the off chance that you value feeling miserable portion of your life. In like manner, I accept you're in a perfect circumstance using either (or a mix) of the going with two intermittent fasting methods.

16/8 Daily Fasting

Ideally, the snappy should then be broken around early evening or by and by in case you wake up at 6-7 take after great numerous individuals. Night times and evenings are commonly spent in the fed state.

To be very genuine, despite the fact that I simply do a submitted brisk once consistently, I apparently do 16/8 snappy – unexpectedly – 2-3 times for every week generally, since I would prefer not to eat anything until about early afternoon.

It doesn't have any kind of effect when you start your 8-hour eating period. You can start at 8 am and stop at 4 pm. Or then again, you start at 2 pm and stop at 10 pm. Do whatever works for you. As a result of my schedule, I will, by and large, eat around 1 pm and 5 pm for the most part days.

The 1-Day Fast

As the name infers, this is a 1-day quick – ordinarily 18-24 hours long.

Here, rather than fasting each day or each other day, you essentially quick once every week. I've seen this as most sensible and maintainable for the vast majority.

To make it simple on yourself, necessarily start your quick after supper so that when you get up the following morning, you've finished around 12 hours of your quick. At that point, if you can make it on the water as well as home grew tea until mid-evening or early night, you're brilliant.

Having trained a large number of individuals through this procedure, let me state that being no picnic for yourself for not making it the full 24 hours is not a smart thought.

Try not to beat yourself up. On the off chance that you've fasted 14, 17, 20, or however numerous hours, simply be content with the way that you've given your body a "breather" to do some truly necessary purifying and mending.

If it's not too much trouble, recollect too that your initial 1-day quick will probably be a test, particularly in case you're accustomed to eating constantly. However, it will likewise be one of the most remunerating encounters you experience as you'll a great deal regarding why you eat.

A lot of times, you'll perceive that you're not ravenous but instead on edge, exhausted, or in a "molded" circumstance (like working at your work area) where you would regularly be eating on nourishment. This mindfulness alone merits doing a 1-day quick.

Whichever sort of intermittent fasting you pick; the extra advantage it gives you is somewhat more adaptable with your diet.

CHAPTER 15:

How to Include and Adapt Intermittent Fasting into Your Lifestyle

This is without a question that a reckless lifestyle is not going to take us anywhere. A lifestyle with no discipline and control would only lead to anarchy. If you don't have a fixed routine, getting up every morning even for a walk can become difficult. People even forget to take their medicines because they don't have a routine for it. Some restrictions are very liberating, and a fixed routine is one among them.

When it comes to health, you can get all kinds of health advice dime a dozen. If you add weight loss as a desired condition, then just the choice of options can be overwhelming. Fitness and wellness have emerged as a very big industry. You can get counseled for dozens of revolutionary procedures for weight loss that seem to work magically on paper and also on the models who never have been fat in the first place. This industry has been in place and thriving for the past few decades and has reached a market valuation of more than $70 billion. Yet. Somehow the obesity has tripled its extent in this world.

Even the weight loss industry, in the end, puts all the blame on the user for not following the process properly.

Not following a lifestyle is not a choice that you can afford. You can follow any kind of lifestyle, but having a healthy lifestyle would always be important.

One of the biggest problems with most lifestyles is that they are very limiting in nature and that's the reason most people are not able to follow them in the long term.

The best thing about intermittent fasting is its sustainability. No matter your line of work or way of living, intermittent fasting can be followed by anyone.

It is a perfect fit for someone living in retirement while also being a perfect match for someone with a hectic traveling job. If you can't spare a lot of money for following a healthy lifestyle then also this lifestyle can be perfect for you or even if you keep your health above everything else, then too this lifestyle can be ideal for you.

It is one lifestyle that can work for you even if you evade exercise initially and would also work if you hate dieting.

The flexibility in almost all the areas is the main forte of intermittent fasting.

Intermittent fasting is a very simple lifestyle focusing on when to eat and not what to eat.

The importance of exercise, diet, sleep and other important aspects of health don't become unwanted in intermittent fasting. They simply bring additional benefits to your results but your results would still come even if you just stick to the intermittent fasting lifestyle.

Intermittent fasting doesn't rely too much on other things to improve your health. It is a simple system to bring your vital functions in sync, and when these things fall into place, other things automatically start arranging themselves in order.

If you exercise, you would naturally lose weight faster, and your health would also improve rapidly. However, even if you are not able to exercise, this doesn't mean that you will not experience weight loss.

The same is the case with diet. Intermittent fasting is a natural way to bring insulin sensitivity. This process helps in reversing several problems in the body. If you follow a healthy keto diet with intermittent fasting, your body can get into ketosis faster. If you don't opt for a keto diet, burning fat would get slow, but natural ketosis would still take place even with a healthy normal diet.

Intermittent fasting is a healthy lifestyle that helps in improving the natural processes of your body. Things like diet, exercise, better sleep routine, etc. will only help improve the results.

It is a very simple lifestyle where you only need to manage two distinct periods of feasting and fasting daily. This is an area in which there can be no major compromise. Everything else in intermittent fasting is adjustable, and we will discuss them in detail.

The ease of following intermittent fasting makes it so sustainable.

The failure of most weight loss methods or lifestyles is that they are difficult to follow in the long run. When you resolve to lose weight or improve your health, you feel very charged and pumped up for the next few days, weeks, and months. However, your resolve starts losing steam as you experience the hardships. The kind of temptation you feel for food on diets. The lethargy and fatigue people feel while doing intense exercises day after day.

Intermittent fasting puts you into so such constraints. The only condition in intermittent fasting is to maintain a fasting period of specified hours. Most of that time will be passed in sleep. Even when you are awake in the last few hours of your fasting window, you know that you will be able to eat after a few hours makes it easier to pass the time.

This is especially important for women over 50 who are trying to adopt a healthy lifestyle as any strict routine will be very difficult to follow in the long run. There is a job, personal life, family, and several other things to balance while juggling all that with a strict routine can be very difficult, and women most of the time choose to stick with their poor routine.

Intermittent fasting would come as a ray of hope in such conditions as you can manage it with any kind of lifestyle and responsibilities. You don't need to prepare extensive meals like in various diets; you don't even need to take out much more time for exercise as you can begin slowly and increase the tempo as you go along the way.

Intermittent fasting is a sustainable way to give your health another big chance and get healthier with minimum effort.

CHAPTER 16:

Food Lists

Your Shopping List

Items on your shopping list should include the following; they are all low on the glycemic index and carry lesser amounts of sugar.

Beverages	Dairy	Meats and Seafood		Vegetables	
Black coffee	1% milk	Canned salmon	Minced beef	Asparagus	Cucumber
Black tea	Almond milk	Canned tuna	Minced pork	Beetroot	Eggplant
Cappuccino with skimmed milk	Fruit yogurt	Chicken liver	Mussels	Bell peppers Bok choy	Kale Leek
Diet coke	Low-fat cottage cheese	Cod	Pre-packed sliced ham	Broccoli	Lettuce (all)
Latte with skimmed milk	Low-fat crème fraiche	Egg	Skinless duck breast	Cabbage	Mushrooms
Lime juice	Low-fat yogurt	Fresh tuna	Skinless chicken breast	Carrot	Red/white onion
Low-calorie hot chocolate	Skim milk	Lean beef	Skinless turkey	Cauliflower	Spinach
Orange squash	Soy milk	Lean ham	Sole	Celery	Tomato
Water	Whole milk	Lean pork	Stewing beef	Chard	Zucchini

Fruit		Sauces, toppings, and dressings	Nuts	Grains and Cereals
Apple	Orange	Basil and tomato sauce	All	Brown rice
Banana	Papaya	Capers	**Seeds**	Bulgur wheat
Blackberries	Peach	Gherkins	All	Couscous
Blueberries	Pear	Jalapeños	**Pulses**	Oats
Cherries	Pineapple	Low-calorie salad dressing	All	Polenta
Cranberries	Plum	Low-fat mayonnaise	**Herbs and spices**	Quinoa
Grapefruit	Raspberries	Olives	All	
Grapes	Strawberries	Pickles	**Fats**	
Kiwi	Tangerine	Pickled onions	Avocado oil	
Lemon	Watermelon	Read-made gravy	Extra-virgin olive oil	
Lime		Red and white vinegar	Grape seed oil	
Melon		Salsa	Sesame seed oil	

Enjoy the Following Foods

Coffee

You won't have to cut the coffee, just skip the lattes and cappuccinos. Coffee is not bad for you; it is how we drink it that affects the body. Choose to drink it with sweetener and low-fat milk rather than with full cream milk and sugar. Coffee is one of the few things people are willing to give up.

Caffeine, the compound found in coffee, is actually why we love the drink so much; it is responsible for numbing the receptors of the brain that make us drowsy, thus making us feel energized. After 15 minutes of drinking a cup, it will begin to work on the brain.

Coffee is also a diuretic (causing the increase of urine production) and is known to impact the digestive system.

Chocolate

Chocolate is not bad for us either, just the choice in chocolate and our willpower that is bad for us. Stay away from white chocolate; it is not real chocolate and opts for darker variants, like 70% cocoa and above. A tad of indulgence is good for you; it boosts your mood too, so have a nibble, but not the whole slab.

Alcohol

Calorie-friendly options include red wine, champagne, gin, and whiskey. Alcohol has the opposite effect on our bodies than caffeine and that is because it tampers our levels of concentration. Whereas coffee peps us up, one drink can wind us down. These effects happen 30 minutes after consuming a glass of bubbles or a drink of choice.

If you are going to have a glass or shot on your fast day, make sure it complies with your calorie count for the day. However, it is best avoided on fasting days.

Nuts

Nuts are satisfying and can help keep the hunger pangs away on the days that you fast. Stick with options such as cashews, almonds, and pistachios. Remember, go easy on the nuts; they are healthy for you but too many can impact your calorie count on fast days. A small handful will do and should help you feel more comfortable if you happen to be struggling with hunger pains.

Seeds

Nibble on larger seeds like a handful of pumpkin seeds or sprinkle raw seeds over salads and roasted vegetables. Sesame and sunflower seeds are popular and are loaded with important vitamins such as zinc, iron, and good fats.

Grains and Cereals

Stick with oats, couscous, brown rice, quinoa, polenta, or bulgur wheat. These foods are low in GI and high in fiber, aiding your digestion and helping you to stay regular. These are important factors when eating healthy and moderating your energy levels.

Herbs and Spices

All are on the green list, so include them wherever you can. They improve the taste of your food. Dishes can be altered by adding a variety of spices and herbs, which may prevent you from getting bored at mealtimes.

Vegetables

Leafy greens such as kale and spinach are your top choices when it comes to your vegetable options, as well as all variants of lettuce too. Green beans are just as healthy for you and are rich in omega-three fatty acids.

Fruit

Stick with your citrus fruits such as lemons, limes, oranges, grapefruit, and tangerines. Certain minerals found in citrus fruits such as grapefruit support the liver by burning fat rather than holding onto it. Be warned though that grapefruit, in particular, can cause contraindications with medications, so check in with your local doctor, especially if you are taking statins. If this does not sound like something you would like to risk, then opt for an apple or a slice of watermelon.

Tomatoes also contain high levels of minerals and nutrients that protect the body from cancers. Munch on an assortment of berries, which are high in antioxidants and rich in vitamin C. Eat all fruits, skin, core, and pips where you can.

Water

Water is necessary for your overall health. Humans lose plenty of it during the day and to maintain an equilibrium, we need to replenish what was lost.

Water does many things; it lends a hand in digestion, allows the nutrients within our bodies to be transported to where they need to be, and aids circulation. All of these things begin to slow down with age.

Most importantly, water affects our skin; being dehydrated causes our skin to become discolored and dry, and are things we wish to avoid as we age.

Foods to Avoid

Added sugar

Skip the fizzy drinks; there are on average eight teaspoons of sugar found in one can of soda. That is a lot when you add up your sugar intake over the whole day. The rule of thumb is to only take in six teaspoons of sugar or less than one ounce over the whole period of the day and even less if you can. This total is made up of the sugar we add to food and the sugar already found in foods.

It is also best to stay away from sweeteners. Sugar occurs in all the food we eat: processed, unprocessed, and naturally occurring like that in milk, honey, fruits, and vegetables.

Did you know the human brain burns sugar? It needs it to function, so it is still a very fundamental part of our livelihood. The "bad" sugars that are usually brought up in diet conversations are those found in sugars and syrups added to processed foods.

When we eat fruits, vegetables, and other natural foods with sugar, we are getting not just the sweetness from them but also all their other, good, whole-some nutrients. When we eat processed foods or add sugar to our cereals and drinks, we are consuming empty calories, which do nothing good for our bodies.

Fats

They are regarded as the worst thing we could consume and tremendously bad for our health and waistlines. **The fats found in food provide twice as many calories as sugars and proteins.** The misconception is that eating "fatty" foods means we are wider and heavier than most, the same as eating a low-fat diet contributing to weight-loss. Obviously, if we combine a low-fat with a restricted calorie intake, weight loss will occur.

Consuming more than what our body needs will make anybody gain weight, regardless of what we eat. If we consume more than what is needed, our body hoards this fat as a fail-safe, so when hunger strikes, we aren't satiated and the body will then feed off this fat storage. A healthy metabolism is there to burn this fat, and less calorie intake means our bodies begin to naturally consume the fat sitting neatly above the waistband of our jeans. Read the packaging and avoid anything with trans-fats at all costs.

Processed Foods

Processed foods are considered a threat to your health, and it is one of the main factors that contribute to illness and obesity.

In general, the majority of the food we eat is processed in some way, shape, or form. For example, butter is created from cream, fruits are plucked from the branches, and meats are minced. There is, however, a stark difference between what has been chemically processed versus mechanically processed.

Consider this rule of thumb: if the item is the sole ingredient found in the jar, without any other chemicals and sugars added, then it is still considered the real deal when it comes to food.

Processed foods are full of empty calories and high in sugars. They are also modified with chemicals to stabilize them and prepare them for the market. These chemicals are also there to ensure longer shelf life too. Flavors are added but not the real thing, making it artificial. These foods also have little to no fiber in them, nor any other benefits.

What makes the whole situation worse is that you can become addicted to processed foods.

CHAPTER 17:

Intermittent fasting and Other Diets

As we now know, intermittent fasting is not exactly a diet, meaning it does not prescribe particular foods or exact amounts of macronutrients. This is why you can generally combine any diet you may be following with intermittent fasting. Of course, if you are following any diet that requires a continuous intake of nutrients you can't fit it in a fasting plan.

But in general, combining your regular diet with intermittent fasting will only mean that you will just keep following your diet, eating what that diet allows and advises you to eat, but you'll just do it during your feeding windows.

Anyway, integration of intermittent fasting with some diets, in particular, may need some extra information due to their own peculiarities. Let's see them in detail.

If you have been trying to lose weight for some time, there is surely a question you have asked yourself more than once: what is the best diet? For decades, scientists, nutritionists, and other food gurus have been throwing away head tackle to decide which diet is most effective for losing weight. High or low in carbohydrates? High or low in fat? Eating three or six times a day? All diets are effective, at least in the short term, because they are based on the same principle: if you expend more calories than you eat, you lose weight.

You may find it hard to believe that calorie restriction is the only proven way to lose weight because you have probably read articles about how fructose, omega 6, toxins, fat, carbohydrates, or gluten are the one absolute culprit of weight gain. But if this is true, some diets would work, and some would not, and I'm sure you have friends who have lost weight with all kinds of diets: high and low fat, high protein, dotted, with supplements, etc.

Unfortunately, although all diets work well at first, most people regain lost weight later. Why?

They are too strict. Reactance is an emotional reaction to prohibition and can increase transgressive behaviors to reaffirm their freedom when the diet restricts our favorite foods, the probability that we pounce on them increases.

They are considered temporary measures, not long-term sustainable changes.

For example, you want to eat a chocolate cookie; you probably would think that since you've already broken the diet, it does it matter to take the whole package, and after that, what's the point have a salad for lunch? Better to give up the day, or the week, or the entire diet.

There are two types of diets: those that restrict amounts and those that restrict food (which, as we pointed out previously, means that they control quantities indirectly).

Intermittent fasting has advantages over both modalities:

Compared to those that reduce quantities: it does not reduce rations during the diet. This produces higher levels of satiety and less sensation of psychological deprivation.

Against those that restrict food (for example, carbohydrates or fats), avoid inadvertently spending calories. With intermittent fasting, you feel less deprived since there are no prohibited foods. On the other hand, losing weight is not the same as losing fat.

Difference with Ketogenic diet

The ketogenic diet and intermittent fasting share huge numbers of similar health benefits since the two methods can have a similar outcome: a condition of ketosis.

Ketosis has many physical and mental benefits, from weight and fat loss to improved feelings of anxiety, mental capacity, and life span. In any case, it's critical to remember that in case you adopt a milder strategy to intermittent keto fasting — for instance, eating inside an 8-hour window — you most likely won't enter ketosis (particularly in the event that you eat a high amount of carbs during that window).

Not everyone who attempts intermittent fasting plans enter ketosis. Indeed, if somebody who fasts also eats high-carb foods, there is a very good chance they will never enter ketosis.

Then again, if ketosis is the objective, you can utilize intermittent keto fasting as an instrument to reach it and improve your overall health.

About biohacking, there most likely are not two more famous practices than the ketogenic high-fat diet and intermittent fasting.

The two regimens have health benefits, including improved digestion, weight loss, and far better immune power.

Ketosis is the process of consuming ketone bodies for energy.

On an ordinary diet, your body consumes glucose as its essential fuel source. Glucose excess is stored as glycogen. At the point when your body is denied glucose (because of exercise, intermittent fasting, or a ketogenic diet), it will go to glycogen for energy. After glycogen is exhausted, will your body begin consuming fat?

A ketogenic diet, which is also called a low-carb, high-fat diet, activates a metabolic move that permits your body to separate fat into ketone bodies in the liver for energy. There are three fundamental ketone bodies found in your blood, pee, and breath:

Acetoacetate: The primary ketone to be made. It can either be changed over into beta-hydroxybutyrate or transformed into $CH_३२CO$ (acetone).

Acetone: Created rapidly from the breakdown of acetoacetate. It is the most unpredictable ketone and is frequently perceptible in the breath when somebody initially goes into ketosis.

Beta-hydroxybutyrate (BHB): This ketone is utilized for energy and the richest in your blood once you are completely in ketosis.

It's additionally the type found in exogenous ketones and it's what ketogenic blood tests measure.

Intermittent Fasting and its relation to Ketosis

Intermittent fasting comprises eating just inside a particular timeframe and not eating for the rest of the hours of the day. Each person, consciously or not, fast overnight from supper to breakfast.

The benefits of fasting have been utilized for a huge number of years in Ayurveda and Traditional Chinese Medicine as an approach to help reset your digestion and help your gastrointestinal framework subsequent to overeating.

As we now know, there are many different ways to deal with intermittent fasting, with different times: (16-20 hours fasting, alternate-day fasting, 24-hour day fasting, and the other we talked about).

Intermittent fasting can put you in a condition of ketosis faster since your cells will rapidly expand your glycogen stores, and afterward begin utilizing your stored fat for fuel.

This prompts an acceleration of the fat-consuming procedure and a ketone levels expansion.

Ketosis and Intermittent Fasting: The Physical Benefits
Both ketogenic diet and intermittent fasting can be excellent tools for:
- Healthy weight loss
- Fat loss without muscle loss
- Balancing cholesterol levels
- Improving insulin effectiveness
- Keeping glucose levels stable

CHAPTER 18:

The Right Mindset to Follow the Diet

This should come as no surprise that most women who pick up a method to lose weight surrender midway. Make no mistake, losing weight is a daunting task, and the body is not ready to give up the fat it loves so dearly.

This means that you can witness periods of no progress. When people are faced with such patches, they lose all the conviction and motivation. They completely stop making an effort and return to their old ways. The result is not hard to guess.

You must understand that losing weight can be hard. You may face several challenges on the way, and there may come several phases when you would want to throw the towel. However, that's the time you need motivation and support.

Finding motivation is very important for the success of any weight loss effort. We all are human beings, and there would be times when you would feel low and would want to give up.

In those times, if there is someone to counsel and provide support, your weight loss journey would get easier.

Usually, this is the toughest thing to do for people trying to lose weight. They fear getting laughed at, ridiculed, or judged. This is a situation that you will have to be prepared for.

Confide in Someone

This is very important that you have someone with whom you can discuss your progress and talk about your efforts. You can confide in your close friend, family members, or anyone else you think would be supportive and understanding. It is not the counseling that one needs in depressing situations but a shoulder to lean on. You can find that shoulder in a friend or family member.

Ensure You Are in a Conducive Environment

This is another important thing that you need to look for. Fasting can be tough at times, and if you are on any specific diet surrounded by people who are eating all the time and specifically eating the things you can't or won't want to eat can be difficult. An easy way out of this problem is to inform your family members about your efforts so that you don't have to face eating people while you are in the fasting period. This lowers the chances of temptation.

Support Groups

Support groups can also be helpful in such efforts. You can join a support group and find other people struggling with similar issues. Such groups can be very helpful in sharing problems and understanding the common impediments that can come in the way.

Support groups help you understand the issues others have faced and that can also ease the pain you may be feeling. Most of the time when we are dealing with a problem and there are no other experiences in front of us as a reference point, our problems start looking very big. The sharing of problems in the support groups helps in building a wider and better perspective.

Seek Professional Help

This is another medium you can use. Several clinics can help you in dealing with the problem, and they can also provide expert guidance in case you are also dealing with other underlying issues.

You can consult clinics that can help in tracking your progress so that staying motivated can become more objective.

Meditation and Positive Affirmations

Meditation is a great way to stay motivated. It is a healthy way to build positive energy inside you and chase away the negative thoughts. Practicing meditation for a few minutes daily can help you in staying motivated.

You can also use positive affirmations to keep yourself motivated. There is scientific evidence behind the fact that repeating positive things can help in driving away stress from the mind, and it makes us feel good. Therefore, if you tend to feel demotivated quickly, taking the help of positive affirmations can be very helpful.

CHAPTER 19:

Exercises to Feel Better for Women Over 50

As with all forms of weight-loss diets, intermittent fasting can only maximize its results if paired with some form of physical exercise. The situation is slightly different when we are talking about individuals over the age of fifty, as the first priority, in this case, will be the overall health of the subject.

What most people fear is the potential of hurting their joints and ligaments, which tend to become more sensible with age. Indeed, this is an underlying factor that cannot be neglected, but it does not exclude all forms of exercise.

When we hear about physical training, the first thought rushed towards the image of a gym, intense workouts and exhaustion. However, people over fifty do not stop working. You might have a physically demanding job, a lifestyle that includes long walks, or even a passion for activities such as yoga.

Although lower on intensity, these are all forms of exercise, ultimately progressing you towards the general goal, burning calories. We do not need to overdo the concept of exercise beyond the point where it gets destructive for our joints, unlike the popular belief that we have to push our bodies to their limits.

There are certain activities that can act as exercise and aid in both the weight loss effects of intermittent fasting and also bring a whole new variety of benefits, such as, but not limited to, preserving joint and ligament health.

Some of these include yoga, as it is not only a light form of exercise, but women, in particular, enjoy the activity on a general basis. You do not need to go to specialized classes in order to engage in this activity, as the internet bears plenty of material regarding art.

Why we do urge you to give yoga classes a try, is the sensation of a group activity, which motivates many and brings more enjoyment to the table. Our main focus is continuity, and if you can find a yoga class where you end up feeling great in the community, this whole process will become even more enjoyable.

Not only that, but most classes have participants with a shared interest, and it should come as no surprise if you happen to stumble upon other women who engage in intermittent fasting, giving you space to share your knowledge in return for more knowledge. The supportive nature of organized classes as well as their popularity; nowadays and the sensation of community make this a great option if you are interested in taking your results to the next level, and perhaps discovering a new hobby.

If you find yoga somehow unfitting for your personal needs, we need to point out another activity that acts in great effect to protect your ligaments, which is swimming.

Swimming is a wonderful sport as it can be done at varying levels of intensity, according to the subject, and aids with preserving joint health and mobility. The question is easy in terms of opportunity; do you enjoy swimming?

If the answer is yes, or you used to enjoy it, going for a few laps once or twice a week will work wonders in terms of boosting your health. It is not overly exhausting, yet provides sufficient stimulus to preserve musculature and keep it safe from the effects of aging long term.

Combined with the number of calories it burns, as well the cardiovascular effects, and this form of mild exercise will be the cornerstone of your health, as it also helps to prevent cardiovascular disease, blood pressure problems, and a variety of muscle, bone and joint issues.

Last but not least, certain gyms feature special classes for people with more advanced age, which focus on light to mild exercises, meant to help you lose weight and preserve muscle and joint health. All of that under the supervision and guidance of a specialized trainer, to make sure all of the workouts are conducted safely.

If neither yoga nor swimming seem attractive to you, this is the last more unique form of physical exercise we have to recommend. Just like with yoga classes, the sensation provided by group workouts and the presence of people similar to you and with share interests can make this environment highly constructive.

As a last mention, if you are uninterested in doing any of the activities listed above, the only small tweak we still have to remind you of is a lot more convenient and milder, yet still effective.

Opting to walk instead of commuting by car or bus whenever possible can make quite a difference, as it burns added calories, mobilizes the legs, and is overall an enjoyable activity.

Fact is, any form of added physical work is going to act in the way you want it to, and as the primary objective is healthy weight loss, we need to focus extensively on the health part.

These activities are amazing for doing just that, and are optimal in order to develop new hobbies, making the weight loss and health-boosting process so much more enjoyable. With that, we are closing this section of the book, with one last idea to mention.

Regular gym workouts under a personal trainer should not be excluded, as most trainers are experienced in working with women over forty or fifty, more than you'd imagine. The downside comes in the cost and intensity these training routines have and are only suitable for people who can preserve the continuity during extended periods of time.

CHAPTER 20:

21-Day (3-Weeks) Meal Plan for 16/8 Method

Week 1

	Monday	Tuesday	Wednesday	Thursday	Friday	Saturday	Sunday
Midnight 4 AM 8 AM	FAST	FAST	FAST	FAST	FAST	FAST	FAST
12 PM	Chocolate Pancakes	Seafood Soup	Fire-Roasted Tomato and Garlic Soup	Breakfast Scramble	Crab Stuffed Mushrooms	Chicken and Prosciutto Spiedini	Oatmeal
4 PM	Coconut Cream with Berries	Curried Tofu Scramble	Pinchos de Pollo Marinated Grilled Chicken Kebabs	Seafood Omelet	Pesto Zucchini Spaghetti	Slow Cooker Bacon and Chicken	Spinach and Pork with Fried Eggs
8 PM Midnight	FAST	FAST	FAST	FAST	FAST	FAST	FAST

Week 2

	Monday	Tuesday	Wednesday	Thursday	Friday	Saturday	Sunday
Midnight 4 AM 8 AM	FAST	FAST	FAST	FAST	FAST	FAST	FAST
12 PM	Smoked Salmon Sandwich	Grilled Cauliflower Steak	Garlic Bacon Wrapped Chicken Bites	Shrimp Deviled Eggs	Broccoli Fried Rice	Smokey Bacon Chicken Meatballs	Scrambles Eggs with Halloumi Cheese
4 PM	Pancakes	Zucchini Green Bean Soup	Asian Chicken Wings	Veggie Omelet	Mexican Cabbage Soup	Baked Garlic Ghee Chicken Breast	Ham Omelet
8 PM Midnight	FAST	FAST	FAST	FAST	FAST	FAST	FAST

Week 3

	Monday	Tuesday	Wednesday	Thursday	Friday	Saturday	Sunday
Midnight 4 AM 8 AM	FAST	FAST	FAST	FAST	FAST	FAST	FAST
12 PM	Savory Breakfast Muffins	Thai Shrimp Soup	Crispy Chicken Thighs	Green Pineapple	Beef & Barley Soup	Chicken and Bacon Sausages	Avocado Egg Bowls
4 PM	Morning Meatloaf	Instant Pot Chicken	Beefsteak Hache (French Hamburgers)	Buttery Date Pancakes	Shrimp Salad	Lemon Ghee Roast Chicken	Low Carb Pancake Crepes
8 PM Midnight	FAST	FAST	FAST	FAST	FAST	FAST	FAST

CHAPTER 21:

21-Day (3-Weeks) Meal Plan for 5:2 Method

Week 1

Day	Breakfast	Lunch	Dinner
Monday (Maximum 500 Calories)	Zucchini Omelet (Calories: 120)	Creamy Southwest Chicken (Calories: 55)	Teriyaki Salmon (Calories: 93)
Tuesday (Eat Normally)	Ham Omelet	Pork Chops with Mushroom Sauce	Sheet Pan Steak Fajitas
Wednesday (Eat Normally)	Chocolate Pancakes	Seafood Soup	Quinoa and Black Bean Casserole
Thursday (Maximum 500 Calories)	Carrot Breakfast Salad (Calories: 50)	Beef Pot Roast (Calories: 64)	Fire-Roasted Tomato and Garlic Soup (Calories: 121)
Friday (Eat Normally)	Breakfast Scramble	Crab Stuffed Mushrooms	Creamy Lamb Korma
Saturday (Eat Normally)	Oatmeal	Pesto Zucchini Spaghetti	Zoodles with White Clam Sauce
Sunday (Eat Normally)	Chia Seed Banana Blueberry Delight	Grilled Cauliflower Steak	Pinchos de Pollo Marinated Grilled Chicken Kebabs

Week 2

Day	Breakfast	Lunch	Dinner
Monday (Maximum 500 Calories)	Crustless Broccoli Sun-dried Tomato Quiche (Calories: 150)	Cheesy Taco Skillet (Calories: 91)	Instant Pot Meatballs (Calories: 103)
Tuesday (Eat Normally)	Coconut Cream with Berries	Zucchini Green Bean soup	Slow Cooker Bacon and Chicken
Wednesday (Eat Normally)	Veggie Omelet	Mexican Cabbage Soup	Garlic Bacon Wrapped Chicken Bites
Thursday (Maximum 500 Calories)	Chili Omelet (Calories: 100)	Thai-Inspired Chicken Salad (Calories: 152)	Chicken and Prosciutto Spiedini (Calories: 174)
Friday (Eat Normally)	Seafood Omelet	Thai Shrimp Soup	Haddock with Spinach and Cauliflower Rice
Saturday (Eat Normally)	Crustless Broccoli Sun-dried Tomato Quiche	Seafood Casserole	
Sunday (Eat Normally)	Savory Breakfast Muffins	Beef & Barley Soup	

Week 3

Day	Breakfast	Lunch	Dinner
Monday (Maximum 500 Calories)	Garlic Zucchini Mix (Calories: 60)	Curried Tofu Scramble (Calories: 114)	Instant Pot Teriyaki Chicken (Calories: 259)
Tuesday (Eat Normally)	Spinach and Pork with Fried Eggs	Instant Pot Chicken	Smokey Bacon Chicken Meatballs
Wednesday (Eat Normally)	Smoked Salmon Sandwich	Shrimp Salad	Asian Chicken Wings
Thursday (Maximum 500 Calories)	Basil and Cherry Tomato Breakfast (Calories: 60)	Broccoli Fried Rice (Calories: 135)	Sheet Pan Chicken and Veggie Bake (Calories: 87)
Friday (Eat Normally)	Shrimp Deviled Eggs	Broccoli Salad	Baked Garlic Ghee Chicken Breast
Saturday (Eat Normally)	Scrambled Eggs with Halloumi Cheese	Shrimp Scampi	Crispy Chicken Thighs
Sunday (Eat Normally)	Pancakes	Southwest Chicken Salad	Chicken and Bacon Sausages

CHAPTER 22:

Breakfast

1. Zucchini Omelet

Preparation Time: 4 minutes
Cooking Time: 3 hours and 30 minutes
Servings: 5
Ingredients:
- 1½ cups red onion, chopped
- 1 tbsp. olive oil
- 2 garlic cloves, minced
- 2 tsp. fresh basil, chopped
- 6 eggs, whisked
- A pinch of sea salt and black pepper
- 8 cups zucchini, sliced
- 6 oz. fresh tomatoes, peeled, crushed

Directions:
1. In a bowl, mix all the ingredients except the oil and the basil.
2. Grease the slow cooker with the oil, spread the omelet mix in the bowl, cover, and cook on low for 3 hours and 30 minutes.
3. Divide the omelet between plates, sprinkle the basil on top, and serve for breakfast.

Nutrition:
- Calories: 35
- Fat: 18 g
- Protein: 15 g
- Carbs: 1.8 g

2. Chili Omelet

Preparation Time: 5 minutes
Cooking Time: 3 hours and 30 minutes
Servings: 5
Ingredients:
- 2 garlic cloves, minced
- 1 tbsp. olive oil
- 1 red bell pepper, chopped
- 1 small yellow onion, chopped
- 1 teaspoon chili powder
- 2 tbsp. tomato puree
- ½ teaspoon sweet paprika
- A pinch of salt and black pepper
- 1 tbsp. parsley, chopped
- 4 eggs, whisked

Directions:
1. In a bowl, mix all the ingredients except the oil and the parsley and whisk them well.
2. Grease the slow cooker with the oil, add the egg mixture, cover, and cook on low for 3 hours and 30 minutes.
3. Divide the omelet between plates, sprinkle the parsley on top, and serve for breakfast.

Nutrition:
- Calories: 33
- Fat: 10 g
- Protein: 15 g
- Carbs: 1.8 g

3. Basil and Cherry Tomato Breakfast

Preparation Time: 4 minutes
Cooking Time: 4 hours
Servings: 20
Ingredients:

- 1 tbsp. olive oil
- 2 yellow onions, chopped
- 2 lb. cherry tomatoes, halved
- 3 tbsp. tomato puree
- 2 garlic cloves, minced
- A pinch of sea salt and black pepper
- 1 bunch basil, chopped

Directions:

1. Grease the slow cooker with the oil, add all the ingredients, cover, and cook on high for 4 hours.
2. Stir the mixture, divide it into bowls and serve for breakfast.

Nutrition:

- Calories: 60
- Fat: 1 g
- Protein: 1 g
- Carbs: 1.8 g

4. Carrot Breakfast Salad

Preparation Time: 5 minutes
Cooking Time: 4 hours
Servings: 2
Ingredients:
- 2 tbsp. olive oil
- 2 lb. baby carrots, peeled and halved
- 3 garlic cloves, minced
- 2 yellow onions, chopped
- ½ cup vegetable stock
- 1/3 cup tomatoes, crushed
- A pinch of salt and black pepper

Directions:
1. In your slow cooker, combine all the ingredients, cover, and cook on high for 4 hours.
2. Divide into bowls and serve for breakfast.

Nutrition:
- Calories: 50
- Fat: 10 g
- Protein: 10 g
- Carbs: 1.8 g

5. Garlic Zucchini Mix

Preparation Time: 5 minutes
Cooking Time: 6 hours
Servings: 5
Ingredients:
- 4 cups zucchinis, sliced
- 2 tbsp. olive oil
- 1 tsp. Italian seasoning
- A pinch of salt and black pepper
- 1 tsp. garlic powder

Directions:
1. In your slow cooker, mix all the ingredients, cover, and cook on low for 6 hours.
2. Divide into bowls and serve for breakfast.

Nutrition:
- Calories: 40
- Fat: 0.7 g
- Protein: 1.5 g
- Carbs: 1.8 g

6. Crustless Broccoli Sun-dried Tomato Quiche

Preparation Time: 4 minutes
Cooking Time: 3 hours and 30 minutes
Servings: 5
Ingredients:

- 12.3-ounce box extra-firm tofu drained and dried
- 1 ½ cup broccoli, chopped
- 2 tsp. yellow mustard
- 1 tbsp. tahini
- 1 tbsp. cornstarch
- ¼ cup old fashioned oats
- ½ tsp. turmeric
- 3-4 dashes of Tabasco sauce
- ½-1 tsp. salt
- ½ cup artichoke hearts, chopped
- 2/3 cup tomatoes, sun-dried, soaked in hot water
- 1/8 cup vegetable broth

Directions:

1. Preheat your oven to 375 degrees Fahrenheit.
2. Prepare a 9" pie plate or springform pan with parchment paper or cooking spray.
3. Put all of the leeks and broccoli on a cookie sheet and drizzle with vegetable broth, salt, and pepper. Bake for about 20-30 min.
4. In the meantime, add the tofu, garlic, nutritional yeast, lemon juice, mustard, tahini, cornstarch, oats, turmeric, salt, and a few dashes of Tabasco in a food processor. When the mixture is smooth, taste for heat and add more Tabasco as needed.
5. Place cooked vegetables with artichoke hearts and tomatoes in a large bowl. With a spatula, scrape in tofu mixture from the processor. Mix carefully, so all of the vegetables are well distributed. If the mixture seems too dry, add a little vegetable broth or water.
6. Add mixture to pie plate muffin tins, or springform pan and spread evenly.
7. Bake for about 35 min. or until lightly browned.
8. Cool before serving. It is delicious, both warm and chilled!

Nutrition:

- Calories: 55
- Fat: 18 g
- Protein: 15 g
- Carbs: 1.8 g

7. Chocolate Pancakes

Preparation Time: 5 minutes
Cooking Time: 80 minutes
Servings: 6
Ingredients:

- 1 ¼ cup gluten-free flour of choice
- 1 tbsp. ground flaxseed
- 1 tbsp. baking powder
- 3 tbsp. nutritional yeast
- 2 tbsp. unsweetened cocoa powder
- ¼ tsp. of sea salt
- 1 cup unsweetened, unflavored almond milk
- 1 tbsp. vegan mini chocolate chips (optional)
- 1 tsp. vanilla extract
- ¼ tsp. stevia powder or 1 tablespoon pure maple syrup
- 1 tbsp. apple cider vinegar
- ¼ cup unsweetened applesauce.

Directions:

1. Get a medium bowl and mix all the dry ingredients (flour, baking powder, flaxseed, cocoa powder, yeast, salt, and optional chocolate chips). Whisk until evenly combined.
2. In a separate small bowl, combine wet ingredients except for the applesauce (almond milk, vanilla extract, apple cider vinegar, maple syrup, or stevia powder).
3. Add wet ingredient mixture and applesauce to the dry ingredients and mix by hand until ingredients are just combined.
4. The batter should sit for 10 minutes. It will rise and thicken, possibly doubling in size.
5. Heat an electric griddle or nonstick skillet to medium heat and spray with a small amount of nonstick spray, if desired. Scoop batter into 3-inch rounds. Much like traditional pancakes, bubbles will start to appear. When bubbles start to burst, flip pancakes and cook for 1-2 minutes. Yields 12 pancakes.

Nutrition:

- Calories: 150
- Fat: 18 g
- Protein: 15 g
- Carbs: 1.8 g

8. Breakfast Scramble

Preparation Time: 5 minutes
Cooking Time: 60 minutes
Servings: 7
Ingredients:

- 1 large head cauliflower, cut up
- 1 seeded, diced green bell pepper
- 1 seeded, diced red bell pepper
- 2 cups sliced mushrooms (approximately 8 oz whole mushrooms)
- 1 peeled, diced red onion
- 3 peeled, minced cloves of garlic
- Sea salt
- 1 ½ tsp. turmeric
- 1–2 tbsp. of low-sodium soy sauce
- ¼ cup nutritional yeast (optional)
- ½ tsp. black pepper

Directions:

1. Sauté green and red peppers, mushrooms, and onion in a medium saucepan or skillet over medium-high heat until onion is translucent (should be 7–8 min). Add an occasional tablespoon or two of water to the pan to prevent vegetables from sticking.
2. Add cauliflower and cook until florets are tenders. It should be 5 to 6 minutes.
3. Add, pepper, garlic, soy sauce, turmeric, and yeast (if using) to the pan and cook for about 5 minutes.

Nutrition:

- Calories: 180
- Fat: 18 g
- Protein: 15 g
- Carbs: 1.8 g

9. Oatmeal

Preparation Time: 5 minutes
Cooking Time: 30 minutes
Servings: 4
Ingredients:
- 1 cup almond milk, unsweetened
- 1 tbsp. Flaxseed, whole
- 1 tbsp. Sunflower seeds
- 1 tbsp. Chia seeds
- 1 ½ tsp. salt

Directions:
1. Dump all of the ingredients together into a small pan and bring the mixture to a boil in a saucepan over medium heat.
2. When it comes to a boil, reduce the heat and allow the mix to simmer gently for two to three minutes until the mix is the desired thickness. Drop a pat of butter on the top and enjoy.

Nutrition:
- Calories 621
- Net carbs 9 g
- Protein 10 g

10. Coconut Cream with Berries

Preparation Time: 5 minutes
Cooking Time: 30 minutes
Servings: 4 Serves
Ingredients:

- 1 ½ cup coconut cream
- 1 tsp. vanilla extract
- 2 oz. strawberries, fresh

Directions:

1. Mix the ingredients together well by using a hand mixer or an immersion mixer if one is available. An added tsp. of coconut oil will increase the amount of fat in this dish.

Nutrition:

- Calories 415
- Net carbs 9 g
- Fat 42 g
- Protein 5 g

11. Seafood Omelet

Preparation Time: 5 minutes
Cooking Time: 30 minutes
Servings: 2
Ingredients:
- 5 oz. shrimp, cooked
- 6 eggs
- 2 tbsp. butter
- 2 tbsp. olive oil
- 1 tbsp. chives, fresh or dried
- 1 ½ cup mayonnaise
- 1 ½ tsp. ground cumin
- ¼ tsp. thyme
- 2 cloves minced garlic
- 1 diced red chili pepper
- ½ tsp. salt
- 1 tsp. white pepper

Directions:
1. Toss the shrimp with olive oil until it is completely covered and fry it gently with the cumin, garlic, salt, chili pepper, and pepper for five minutes.
2. While the shrimp mix cools beat the eggs and pours them into the skillet. Let the eggs sit undisturbed while they cook until the edges begin to brown and the center has mostly set firm. Then add the chives and the mayonnaise to the shrimp mixture.
3. Pour the shrimp mixture onto the egg that is frying in the skillet and fold the omelet in half, frying for an additional three minutes on each side.

Nutrition:
- Calories 872
- Net carbs 4 g
- Fat 83 g
- Protein 27 g

12. Spinach and Pork with Fried Eggs

Preparation Time: 5 minutes

Cooking Time: 30 minutes

Servings: 2

Ingredients:
- 2 cups baby spinach
- 6 oz. pork loin, smoked, cut into chunks
- 4 eggs
- ½ tsp. salt
- 1 tsp. black pepper
- ¼ cup chopped walnuts
- ¼ cup frozen cranberries
- 3 tbsp. butter

Directions:
1. Wash, dry, and chop the baby spinach. Fry the spinach in the butter for five minutes stirring continuously. Remove the spinach from the pan and let it drain on a paper towel. Fry the chunks of pork loin in the same skillet for five minutes.
2. Remove the pork from the skillet and then put the cooked baby spinach back in, adding the nuts and cranberries. Stir constantly while this is cooking for five minutes.
3. Pour the mix into a bowl. Fry the eggs and place two on each plate with half of the spinach mixture. Serve with the chunks of fried pork loin.

Nutrition:
- Calories 1033
- Net carbs 8 g
- Fat 99 g
- Protein 26 g

13. Smoked Salmon Sandwich

Preparation Time: 5 minutes
Cooking Time: 30 minutes
Servings: 2
Ingredients:
TOPPING

- 4 eggs - 1 tbsp. chives, fresh, chop
- 3 oz. smoked salmon
- 2 tbsp. heavy whipping cream
- ½ tsp. salt
- ½ tsp. white pepper
- 1 oz. chop fine kale
- 2 tbsp. butter
- ¼ tsp. chili powder - 2 tbsp. olive oil

SPICY PUMPKIN BREAD

- 1 tbsp. lard - 14 oz. pure pumpkin
- 25 cups coconut oil - 3 eggs
- 1/3 cup seeds pumpkin - 1/3 cup chopped walnuts
- 1 tbsp. baking powder - 2 tbsp. pie spice pumpkin
- ½ cup flaxseed - 1 ¼ cups coconut flour
- 1 ¼ cups almond flour
- 2 tbsp. psyllium husk powder, ground - 1 tsp. salt

Directions:

1. Heat oven to 400. Use the lard to grease a nine by nine pan. Add the baking powder, pumpkin pie spice, nuts, psyllium husk powder, flaxseed, both flours, salt, and seeds into a bowl and mix together well. Use a separate bowl to cream together the oil, pumpkin puree, and egg. Gently pour this mixture into the dry ingredients and fold both together until all of the ingredients are well moistened. Spoon this entire mixture into the greased baking pan and bake it for one hour. Allow the bread to cool completely.
2. When the bread is done beat together the cream and eggs with the pepper and salt. Scramble the egg mix in the melted butter for five minutes, stirring constantly, and then mix in the chili powder. Slice off two slices of the pumpkin bread and place them in the toaster to toast for three minutes. Butter the toasted pumpkin bread and lay each slice on a plate. Top each slice with the kale and the smoked salmon. Place the eggs on top of this and sprinkle with the chives.

Nutrition:

- Calories 678 Net carbs 3 g Fat 55 g Protein 41 g

14. Shrimp Deviled Eggs

Preparation Time: 5 minutes
Cooking Time: 30 minutes
Servings: 4
Ingredients:
- 1 tsp. chopped chives
- ¼ cup mayonnaise
- 4 hard-boiled eggs
- 8 fresh sprigs dill
- 1 tsp. Tabasco sauce
- 8 larges fully cooked, peeled and deveined shrimp
- ½ tsp. salt
- ½ tsp. white pepper

Directions:
1. Carefully peel the chilled hard-boiled eggs and then cut them in half the long way and remove the yolks. Put the yolks into a bowl and use a dinner fork to gently mash the yolks and then add the Tabasco, salt, and mayonnaise. Mix all of this together well and then carefully spoon the mixture back into the egg whites. Top each egg with one cooked shrimp and a sprig of dill.
2. *Shrimp are sold whole or peeled and deveined. You can peel them yourself and remove the vein but the cost difference to buy them already peeled and deveined (P & D) is very small and worth the price.

Nutrition:
- Calories 163
- Net carbs 5 g
- Fat 15 g
- Protein 7 g

15. Scrambled Eggs with Halloumi Cheese

Preparation Time: 5 minutes
Cooking Time: 30 minutes
Servings: 2
Ingredients:

- 4 eggs
- 4 slices bacon
- ½ tsp. salt
- 1 tsp. black pepper
- ¼ tsp. chili powder
- ½ cup black olives, pitted if needed
- ½ cup parsley, fresh, chopped fine
- 2 scallions
- 2 tbsp. olive oil
- 3 oz. halloumi cheese, diced from a block

Directions:

1. Chop finely the bacon and the cheese. Fry the bacon and the cheese with the scallions in olive oil for five minutes. While this mixture is frying beat the eggs well with the parsley, pepper, chili powder, and salt. Dump the egg mix onto the bacon cheese mix in the skillet and scramble all together for three minutes while stirring constantly. Add in the olives and cook for three more minutes.

Nutrition:

- Calories 667
- Carbs 4 g
- Fat 59 g
- Protein 28 g

16. Pancakes

Preparation Time: 5 minutes
Cooking Time: 15 minutes
Servings: 2
Ingredients:
- 1 large egg
- 2 white eggs
- 2 tbsp. cream cheese
- 3 tbsp. unsweetened, canned pumpkin (not pie filling)
- 1 tbsp. vanilla extract
- 2/3 cup almond flour
- 2 tbsp. coconut flour
- 1 tbsp. swerve Sweetener.
- 1 tsp. pumpkin pie spice
- 1/8 tsp. salt
- 1 tsp. baking powder
- ¼ tsp. baking soda - ½ tsp. xanthan gum
- Water as needed

Topping:
- 1/3 cup cream cheese - 2 tbsp. unsweetened canned pumpkin
- 1 to 1 ½ tbsp. swerve sweetener
- ½ tsp. cinnamon - 1/8 tsp. pumpkin pie spice
- ½ tsp. vanilla extract

Direction:
1. Preheat a griddle to 350°F and spray with non-stick cooking spray.
2. Add all the wet pancake ingredients except water into a blender and blend. Then add the dry ingredients and blend until smooth. Add water a little at a time until the pancake batter has the right consistency. Pour a small amount of batter onto a heated griddle.
3. Cook until browned and the edges (almost to the center) are dry for about 3 to 4 minutes.
4. Then flip and cook for 2 to 3 minutes more.
5. For the topping: in a processor, add all topping ingredients and blend until creamy.
6. Top the pancakes with toppings and drizzle with maple syrup.

Nutrition:
- Calories 206 Total Fat 14.4 g
- Cholesterol 73 mg Sodium 289 mg
- Total Carbohydrate 11 g
- Protein 7.6 g

17. Veggie Omelet

Preparation Time: 7 minutes
Cooking Time: 10 minutes
Servings: 2
Ingredients:
- 3 eggs
- 1 tbsp. almond milk or water
- ½ tsp. salt kosher
- ½ tsp. freshly ground black pepper
- 3 tbsp. unsalted butter
- 1 bunch Swiss chard, cleaned and stemmed
- 1/3 cup Ricotta

Directions:
1. Crack the eggs in a bowl. Add water or milk, season with salt and pepper. Whisk it using a fork and keep it aside. Melt 2 tbsp. butter over medium-high heat in an 8-inch nonstick skillet. Add a few of the Swiss chard and continue to sauté until just wilted.
2. Remove from pan. Set aside. Melt 1 tbsp. butter in the skillet. Then slowly add the egg mixture and tilt the pan, so the mixture spreads evenly. Allow the egg to firm up a bit. Cook for another 1 minute.
3. Spoon in the ricotta when the edges are firm, but the center is still a bit runny. With a spatula, fold about 1/3 of the omelet over the ricotta filling. Serve on a plate with Swiss chard.

Nutrition:
- Calories 652
- Total Fat 57.9 g
- Cholesterol 608 mg
- Sodium 1776 mg
- Total Carbohydrate 8.2 g
- Protein 27.5 g

18. Ham Omelet

Preparation Time: 10 minutes
Cooking Time: 5 minutes
Servings: 2
Ingredients:
- 1 ½ tbsp. unsalted butter
- 10 eggs
- 2 tbsp. milk
- 1 tsp. kosher salt
- ¼ tsp. freshly ground black pepper
- 1 ¼ cups cooked ham
- 1 ½ cups diced Shredded sharp cheddar
- 1/3 cup chopped fresh chives

Directions:
1. Melt the butter in a skillet. Add ham and sauté until browned. Meanwhile, whisk together the eggs, pepper, kosher salt, and milk in a bowl.
2. Pour into the pan and cook for 4 to 5 minutes, or until the desired doneness. Stirring occasionally. Just before the eggs are set, add chives and cheddar.

Nutrition:
- Calories 175
- Total Fat 9.4 g
- Cholesterol 38 mg
- Sodium 1084 mg
- Total Carbohydrate 3.1 g
- Protein 19 g

19. Savory Breakfast Muffins

Preparation Time: 20 minutes
Cooking Time: 25 minutes
Servings: 2
Ingredients:
- 8 eggs
- 1 cup shredded cheese
- Salt and pepper to taste
- ½ tsp. baking powder
- ¼ cup diced onion
- 2/3 cup coconut flour
- 1 ½ cup spinach
- ¼ cup full fat coconut milk
- 1 tbsp. basil, chopped
- ½ cup cooked chicken, diced finely

Directions:
1. Preheat the oven to 375°F. Use butter or oil to grease your muffin tray or you can use muffin paper liners. In a large mixing bowl, whisk the eggs.
2. Add in the coconut milk and mix again. Gradually shift in the coconut flour with baking powder salt. Add in the cooked chicken, onion, spinach, basil, and combine well. Add the cheese and mix again. Pour the mixture onto your muffin liners. Bake for about 25 minutes. Serve at room temperature.

Nutrition:
- Calories 388
- Fat 25.8 g
- Carbohydrate 8.6 g
- Proteins 25.3 g

20. Green Pineapple

Preparation Time: 5 minutes

Cooking Time: 0 minutes

Servings: 2

Ingredients:
- ½ of a pineapple
- 1 broccoli, diced
- 1 cup of water
- 1 long cucumber, diced
- A dash of salt
- 1 kiwi, diced

Directions:
1. Add kiwi, cucumber, pineapple, broccoli, and water in a blender. Add the salt and blend until smooth. Serve.

Nutrition:
- Calories 251
- Fats 0.4 g
- Proteins 0.5 g
- Carbohydrates 22 g

21. Avocado Egg Bowls

Preparation Time: 15 minutes
Cooking Time: 5 minutes
Servings: 2
Ingredients:
- 1 tsp. coconut oil
- 2 organics, free-range Salt and pepper
- 1 Large & ripe avocado
- For Garnishing:
- Chopped walnuts
- Balsamic Pearls
- Fresh thyme

Directions:
1. Slice your avocado in two, then take out the pit and remove enough of the inside so there is enough space inside to accommodate an entire egg.
2. Cut off a little bit of the bottom of the avocado so the avocado will sit upright as you place it on a stable surface. Open your eggs and put each of the yolks in a separate bowl or container. Place the egg whites in the same small bowl. Sprinkle some pepper and salt into the whites, according to your taste, then mix them well.
3. Melt the coconut oil in a pan that has a lid that fits and put it on med-high. Put in the avocado boats, with the meaty side down on the pan, the skin side up, and sauté them for approx. 35 seconds, or when they become darker in color.
4. Turn them over, then add to the spaces inside, almost filling the inside with the whites of the eggs. Then, reduce the temperature and place the lid. Let them sit covered it for approx. 16 to 20 minutes until the whites are just about fully cooked.
5. Gently add one yolk onto each of the avocados and keep cooking them for 4 to 5 mins, just until they get to the point of cook you want them at. Move the avocados to a dish and add toppings to each of them using the walnuts, the balsamic pearls, or/and thyme.

Nutrition:
- Calories 215
- Fat 18 g
- Carbohydrates 8 g
- Protein 9 g

22.   Morning Meatloaf

Preparation Time: 30 minutes
Cooking Time: 25 minutes
Servings: 2
Ingredients: (6 Servings)
- 1 ½ pound of breakfast sausage
- 6 large organic eggs
- 2 tbsp. of unsweetened non-dairy milk
- 1 small onion, finely chopped
- 2 medium garlic cloves, peeled and minced
- 4 oz. of cream cheese softened and cubed
- 1 cup of shredded cheddar cheese
- 3 tbsp. of scallions, finely chopped
- 1 cup of water at room temperature.

Directions:
1. Add all the ingredients apart from water in a large bowl. Stir until well combined. Form the sausage mixture into a meatloaf and wrap it with a sheet of aluminum foil. Make sure your meat left fits into the pot properly. If not, remove parts of the mixture and reserve them for future use. Once you wrap the meatloaf into a packet, add 1 cup of water and a trivet to your Instant Pot. Put the meatloaf on the trivet's top. Cover and cook for 25 minutes on high pressure. When done, quickly release the pressure. Carefully remove the lid. Unwrap the meatloaf and check if the meatloaf is done. Serve and enjoy!

Nutrition:
- Calories 592
- Carbohydrates 2.5 g
- Proteins 11 g
- Fats 49.5 g

23. Buttery Date Pancakes

Preparation Time: 10 minutes
Cooking Time: 10 minutes
Servings: 2
Ingredients:

- ¼ cup almond flour
- 3 eggs, beaten
- 1 tsp. olive oil
- 6 dates, pitted
- 1 tbsp. almond butter
- 1 tsp. vanilla extract
- ½ tsp. ground cinnamon

Directions:

1. Stir the eggs in a bowl make them fluffy.
2. Wash the dates and cut them in half.
3. Discard the seeds and mash them finely.
4. Melt the almond butter and add to the eggs.
5. Add the almond flour, olive oil and cinnamon.
6. Mix well and add the vanilla extract.
7. Mix into a smooth batter.
8. Add the date paste and mix well.
9. In a pan heat the butter over medium heat.
10. Add the butter using a spoon and fry them golden brown from both sides.
11. Repeat with all the batter.
12. Serve with melted butter on top.

Nutrition:

- Calories 281
- Fat 20 g
- Protein 10.5 g
- Carbohydrates 4.5 g

24.   Low Carb Pancake Crepes

Preparation Time: 10 minutes
Cooking Time: 10 minutes
Servings: 2
Ingredients:

- 3 oz. cream cheese
- 1 tsp. ground cinnamon
- 1 tbsp. honey
- 1 tsp. ground cardamom
- 1 tsp. butter
- 2 beaten eggs

Directions:

1. In a bowl, whisk the eggs finely.
2. Beat the cream cheese in a different bowl until it becomes soft.
3. Add the egg mixture to the softened cream cheese and mix well until there are no lumps left.
4. Add cinnamon, cardamom, and honey to it. Mix well. The butter would be runnier than pancake batter.
5. In a pan add the butter and heat over medium heat.
6. Add the butter using a scooper, that way all the sizes of the crepes would be the same.
7. Fry them golden brown on both sides.
8. Repeat the process with the rest of the butter.
9. Drizzle some honey on top and enjoy.

Nutrition:

- Calories 241
- Fats 21.8 g
- Carbohydrates 2.4 g
- Proteins 9.6 g

25. Chia Seed Banana Blueberry Delight

Preparation Time: 30 minutes
Cooking Time: 0 minutes
Servings: 2

Ingredients:

- 1 cup yogurt
- ½ cup blueberries
- ½ tsp. Salt
- ½ tsp. Cinnamon
- 1 banana
- 1 tsp. Vanilla Extract
- ¼ cup Chia Seeds

Directions:

1. Discard the skin of the banana.
2. Cut into semi-thick circles.
3. You can mash them or keep them as a whole if you like to bite into your fruits.
4. Clean the blueberries properly and rinse well.
5. Soak the chia seeds in water for 30 minutes or longer.
6. Drain the chia seeds and transfer them into a bowl.
7. Add the yogurt and mix well.
8. Add the salt, cinnamon and vanilla, and mix again.
9. Now fold in the bananas and blueberries gently.
10. If you want to add dried fruit or nuts, add it and then serve immediately.
11. This is best served cold.

Nutrition:

- Calories 260
- Fats 26.6 g
- Carbohydrates 17.4 g
- Protein 4.1 g

CHAPTER 23:

Lunch

26. Cheesy Taco Skillet

Preparation time: 10 minutes
Cooking time: 25 minutes
Servings: 12
Ingredients:
- 1 lb. lean ground beef
- 1 large yellow onion, diced
- 2 bell peppers, diced
- 1 can diced tomatoes with green chilis
- Taco seasoning, to taste
- 3 cups baby kale mixture
- 1 1/2 cup cheddar cheese, shredded
- Green onions, to garnish

Direction:
1. Take a large-sized pan and place it over medium heat.
2. Lightly grease the pan with cooking spray.
3. Add ground beef to the pan and stir-fry until brown.
4. Add peppers, onions and sauté until golden brown in color.
5. Add taco seasoning, canned tomatoes and a splash of water, then mix well.
6. Toss in greens and cook until they are wilted.
7. Stir in shredded cheese and cook until the cheese is melted.
8. Transfer the beef and cheese mixture to the serving plate.
9. Serve fresh with your favorite garnish.
10. Enjoy.

Nutrition:
- Calories 91 Total Fat 14.2g
- Saturated Fat 7.7g Carbohydrate 10.7g
- Dietary Fiber 1.6g
- Sugars 3.2g
- Protein 29.5g

27. Pork Chops with Mushroom Sauce

Preparation time: 20 minutes
Cooking time: 30 minutes
Servings: 20
Ingredients:

- 4 boneless pork chops
- Kosher salt, to taste
- Ground black pepper, to taste
- 2 tablespoons olive oil
- 8 oz. baby Bella mushrooms, sliced
- 2 garlic cloves, minced
- 1/2 cup heavy cream
- 1/2 cup freshly grated Parmesan
- 1 teaspoon dried oregano
- Pinch crushed red pepper flakes
- 3 cups packed baby spinach

Direction:

1. Place the pork chops on a working surface and pat them dry with a paper towel.
2. Drizzle salt and black pepper over both sides of the pork chops and rub them well.
3. Leave the pork chops at room temperature for 5 minutes.
4. Take a large-sized skillet and place it over medium heat.
5. Add oil to the skillet and sear the pork chops in the hot oil.
6. Cook each pork chop for 6-8 minutes per side until golden brown.
7. Once the pork chops are completely cooked, transfer them to a plate.
8. Cover the seared chops with another plate and keep them warm.
9. Add mushrooms to the same skillet and sauté for 5 minutes.
10. Stir in garlic and stir-fry for 1 minute.
11. Add oregano, red pepper flakes, Parmesan and heavy cream to the mushrooms.
12. Mix well and adjust the mushroom's seasoning with salt and black pepper.
13. Cook the sauce for 3 minutes approximately until it thickens.
14. Toss in spinach leaves and cook for 2 minutes until they are wilted.
15. Place the seared pork chops back in the skillet with the sauce and cook for 5 minutes until heated.
16. Serve warm and fresh.

Nutrition:

- Calories 65 Total Fat 4.11g Saturated Fat 1.4g Carbohydrate 10.94g Dietary Fiber 2.2g
- Sugars 0.61g Protein 11.22g

28. Beef Pot Roast

Preparation time: 20 minutes
Cooking time: 6 hours, 24 minutes
Servings: 10
Ingredients:

- 1 (3 lbs.) beef pot roast
- Salt and black pepper, to taste
- 1 tablespoon coconut flour

Mushroom Sauce:

- 2 tablespoons vegetable oil
- 8 oz. mushrooms, sliced
- 1 onion, chopped
- 2 garlic cloves, minced
- 1 tablespoon butter
- 1 1/2 tablespoons almond flour
- 1 tablespoon tomato paste
- 2 1/2 cups chicken broth
- 3 medium carrots, diced - 2 stalks celery, diced
- 1 sprig fresh rosemary - 2 sprigs fresh thyme

Direction:

1. Place the beef pot roast on the working surface and pat it dry with a paper towel.
2. Drizzle salt, black pepper and flour over the roast and rub it all over the meat.
3. Take a large-sized skillet and place it over medium-high heat.
4. Pour vegetable oil into the skillet and add the beef pot roast to sear.
5. Cook each side of the roast for 6 minutes until well cooked. Remove the roast from the skillet and keep it on a plate, covered and warm. Reduce the heat of the skillet to medium and add mushrooms and butter. Sauté for approximately 4 minutes, then add the onion.
6. Stir-fry for another 5 minutes until the onions are soft.
7. Add garlic and cook, stirring for 1 minute. Gently add 1 ½ tablespoon flour and cook for 1 minute. Stir in tomato paste and cook for another minute.
8. Pour in chicken broth and cook, stirring to a simmer.
9. Transfer the sauce to a slow cooker, then add carrots, celery, roast, vegetables, rosemary, and thyme. Cover the roast and cook for 6 hours on high heat. Adjust the sauce's seasoning with salt and black pepper. Slice the roast and serve warm.

Nutrition per serving:

- Calories 64 Total Fat 19.3g Saturated Fat 7.7g Carbohydrate 4.8g Dietary Fiber 1.9g
- Sugars 2.4g Protein 23.5g

29. Creamy Southwest Chicken

Preparation time: 10 minutes
Cooking time: 20 minutes
Servings: 7
Ingredients:
- 1 tablespoon olive oil
- 2 chicken breast, boneless, skinless
- ¼ cup onion, minced
- 2 garlic cloves, minced
- 4 ½ oz. can green chilis, chopped
- 1/4 cup heavy cream
- 1/4 cup cheddar cheese, shredded

Direction:
1. Place the chicken on the working surface and pat it dry with a paper towel.
2. Dice the chicken into small bite-sized pieces.
3. Season the pieces with salt and black pepper.
4. Take a large-sized skillet and place it over medium heat.
5. Add oil to the skillet and let it heat.
6. Toss in the chicken pieces and sear until golden brown.
7. Add onions and cook until soft then add garlic.
8. Stir-fry 1 minute and add cream and green chilis.
9. Cook the mixture on a simmer until it thickens.
10. Top the chicken mixture with shredded cheddar cheese.
11. Cook until the cheese is melted.
12. Serve warm and fresh.

Nutrition:
- Calories 55
- Total Fat 11.1 g
- Saturated Fat 4.3 g
- Carbohydrate 2.4 g
- Dietary Fiber 0.2 g
- Sugars 1.3 g
- Protein 26.1 g

30. Seafood Casserole

Preparation time: 30 minutes
Cooking time: 35 minutes
Servings: 12
Ingredients:
Poached Seafood:
- 1 cup dry white wine - 1 cup water
- 2 small bay leaves, whole - 1/2 teaspoon old bay seasoning
- oz. shrimp, thawed, peeled and deveined - 12 oz. cod, diced

Vegetables: 2 stalks celery, diced - 2 tablespoons butter
- 2 medium leeks, white part only, sliced - Sea salt, to taste

Sauce:
- 1/2 teaspoon xanthan gum - 1 cup heavy whipping cream
- 1 tablespoon butter - 1/4 teaspoon sea salt

Topping:
- 1 tablespoon butter - 4 oz. Parmesan cheese, shredded - 2 teaspoons old bay seasoning
- 1/4 cup almond flour - 1 tablespoon fresh parsley, chopped

Direction:
1. Set the oven's temperature at 400 degrees F to preheat. Take a large-sized saucepan and place it over medium-high heat. Add dry white wine, bay leaves, water, and ½ teaspoon old bay to the saucepan. Cook the mixture for 3 minutes on a simmer. Add shrimp to the wine mixture and cook until the shrimp changes color.
2. Remove the shrimp from the poaching liquid using a slotted spoon and transfer to a plate. Add cod to the poaching liquid and cook until the fish turns white. Remove the codfish from the liquid and keep it aside on a plate.
3. Cook the poaching liquid until it is reduced to 1 cup. Take a Dutch oven and place it over medium-high heat. Add 2 tablespoons butter to the Dutch oven and melt it. Stir in leeks and celery then stir-fry until soft. Season the vegetables with sea salt, then remove from heat. Spread the vegetables in a casserole dish, then toss in the seafood.
4. Add sauce ingredients to the same Dutch oven and cook, stirring until it thickens.
5. Pour the sauce over the seafood in the casserole dish.
6. Prepare the topping by blending almond flour with 1 tablespoon butter, 2 teaspoons old bay and Parmesan cheese. Spread this crumble over the seafood mixture then bake for 20 minutes in the oven. Serve warm and fresh.

Nutrition:
- Calories 62 Total Fat 12.9g Saturated Fat 7.7g Carbohydrate 3.6g Dietary Fiber 0.1g
- Sugars 0.5g Protein 32.5g

31. Shrimp Scampi

Preparation time: 20 minutes
Cooking time: 12 minutes
Servings: 9

- Ingredients:
- 1 ¼ pound shrimp, peeled and deveined
- 4 tablespoons butter
- 3 garlic cloves, roughly chopped
- 1/4 cup Chardonnay
- 1/4 cup lemon juice
- 1/4 teaspoon red pepper flakes
- 1/4 cup parsley, chopped
- 2 scallions, sliced
- 1/2 cup shredded Parmesan cheese
- Salt and black pepper, to taste
- oz. cherry tomatoes, halved

Direction:

1. Peel and devein the shrimp and keep them ready aside.
2. Finely chop the parsley and garlic.
3. Take a large-sized sauté pan and place it over medium heat.
4. Add butter to the pan and heat it to melt.
5. Stir in garlic and sauté until soft.
6. Toss in shrimp and stir-fry until they turn pink.
7. Flip the shrimp and season with red pepper flakes.
7. Add lemon juice and wine, then cook until the liquid is reduced.
8. Remove the shrimp from heat and add parsley.
9. Garnish with Parmesan and serve warm.

Nutrition:

- Calories :70
- Total Fat 10 g
- Saturated Fat 5.8 g
- Carbohydrate 5.5 g
- Dietary Fiber 0.9 g
- Sugars 2.6 g
- Protein 23.2 g

32. Seafood Soup

Preparation time: 15 minutes
Cooking time: 35 minutes
Servings: 6
Ingredients:
Soup:

- 2 tablespoons olive oil
- 1 white onion, chopped
- 2 garlic cloves, crushed
- cups fish broth
- 1 cup white wine
- 1 bay leaf
- 3 tomatoes, peeled, deseeded, and chopped
- 1 teaspoon salt
- 9 oz. white fish
- 20 shrimps - 16 fresh mussels
- 8 scallops
- 1/3 oz. fresh thyme, to garnish
- ½ lime, sliced, to garnish

Garlic mayo:

- 1 egg - 1 garlic clove - ½ lemon, the juice
- ¼ teaspoon salt - 1 cup olive oil

Direction:

1. Take a large-sized soup pot and place it over medium heat.
2. Add olive oil to the soup pot and let it heat. Toss in onions and sauté until soft and translucent. Stir in crushed garlic and cook until golden brown.
3. Add white wine, fish broth, salt, tomatoes, and bay leaf.
4. Cook the mixture to a boil first, then reduce the heat to a simmer.
5. Continue cooking for 25 minutes until it forms a smooth gravy.
6. Meanwhile, prepare the garlic mayonnaise by adding egg, lemon juice, garlic clove, and salt to a small blender. Blend mayonnaise ingredients well until smooth and white in color. Add mussels, scallops and fish fillets then cook for another 3 minutes.
7. Garnish the soup with lime slices and fresh thyme. Serve warm with a dollop of garlic mayonnaise on top. Enjoy.

Nutrition per serving:

- Calories 345 Total Fat 25.9 g Saturated Fat 4.3 g Carbohydrate 6.2 g
- Dietary Fiber 0.9 g Sugars 2.1g Protein 28 g

33. Crab Stuffed Mushrooms

Preparation time: 20 minutes
Cooking time: 25 minutes
Servings: 4
Ingredients:

- oz. fresh crab meat
- 1 lb. cremini mushrooms, cleaned and destemmed
- 3 garlic cloves, minced
- oz. cream cheese, softened
- 1/3 cup sharp cheddar cheese, shredded
- ½ cup Parmesan cheese, shredded
- ¼ cup sour cream
- Sea salt and black pepper, to taste
- 3 green onions, chopped
- 1 tablespoon Dijon mustard
- Cooking oil

Direction:

1. Set the oven's temperature to 400 degrees F to preheat.
2. Take a rimmed baking sheet and layer its bottom with parchment paper.
3. Place the mushroom caps in the baking sheet and brush them with cooking oil.
4. Bake the mushroom caps for 10 minutes in the preheated oven.
5. Meanwhile, take a large mixing bowl and add crab, cream cheese, cheddar cheese, green onions, garlic, sour cream, salt, black pepper, and Dijon mustard.
6. Mix the crab mixture well, then divide it in the mushroom caps.
7. Bake the mushrooms again for 10 minutes approximately.
9. Drizzle Parmesan cheese over the stuffed mushrooms.
10. Return them to the oven and bake again for 5 minutes until the cheese is golden brown.
11. Garnish with freshly chopped herbs.
12. Serve warm.

Nutrition:

- Calories 399 Total Fat 25.4 g
- Saturated Fat 15.4g Carbohydrate 16.8 g
- Dietary Fiber 4 g
- Sugars 7.5 g
- Protein 29.7 g
- Vegan

34. Curried Tofu Scramble

Preparation time: 20 minutes
Cooking time: 23 minutes
Servings: 2
Ingredients:
Scramble:

- 3 tablespoons vegetable broth
- ½ medium onion, chopped
- 1 large red pepper, diced
- oz. mushrooms, sliced
- ½ block extra-firm tofu, pressed and drained
- 3 cups greens, chopped
- Curry Seasoning:
- ½ teaspoon cumin
- 1 tablespoon water
- ¼ teaspoon coriander powder
- ½ teaspoon curry powder
- ½ teaspoon garlic powder
- ¼ teaspoon turmeric powder
- ¼ teaspoon garam masala
- ¼ teaspoon paprika
- ¼ teaspoon black salt

Direction:

1. Take a large-sized pan and place it over medium heat.
2. Add vegetable broth and onions to the pan and cook for 5 minutes.
3. Stir diced red peppers and mushrooms, then cook for 10 minutes with occasional stirring.
4. Push the cooked veggies to the side of the cooking pan and place the pressed tofu block in the center. Cook the tofu for 3 minutes while breaking it into chunks.
5. Meanwhile, add the seasonings and spices to a small bowl.
6. Mix the spices well then sprinkle over the tofu to season it.
7. Toss well until the tofu crumbles are thoroughly mixed with the seasonings.
8. Place the greens over the tofu and immediately cover with the lid.
9. Let it cook for 5 minutes on low heat until the greens are wilted.
10. Garnish the tofu scramble with green onions and hot sauce. Serve warm.

Nutrition:

- Calories 114 Total Fat 2.8 g Saturated Fat 0.5 g Carbohydrate 17.9 g
- Dietary Fiber 5.7 g Sugars 6.8g Protein 8.9 g

35. Pesto Zucchini Spaghetti

Preparation time: 30 minutes
Cooking time: 12 minutes
Servings: 2
Ingredients:

- cherry tomatoes, halved
- 1/3 cup vegan pesto
- 1/2 red onion, thinly sliced and halved
- 2 medium zucchinis, spiralized
- mushrooms, thinly sliced
- 2 cloves garlic, finely minced
- Salt, to taste
- Ground black pepper, to taste
- 2 teaspoons olive oil
- Red crushed pepper, to taste
- Cashew cream, to serve

Direction:

1. Take a nonstick pan and place it over medium-high heat.
2. Add olive oil to the pan along with sliced mushrooms, sliced onions, and minced garlic.
3. Adjust seasoning with ¼ teaspoon salt and mix well.
4. Sauté the vegetables for 5 minutes or more until the veggies are soft.
5. Transfer the cooked vegetables to a plate and keep them warm.
6. Wipe the pan with a paper towel and place it over medium heat.
7. Add ¼ cup pesto and spiralized zucchini to the pan and stir-fry for 2 minutes.
8. Immediately transfer the zucchini to a suitable bowl.
9. Add sautéed veggies to the zucchini spaghetti along with cherry tomatoes.
10. Toss the ingredients well with the zucchini.
11. Add the rest of the pesto and cashews cream.
12. Mix again and adjust the spaghetti seasoning with salt, black pepper, and red crushed pepper.
13. Serve warm and fresh.

Nutrition:

- Calories 206 Total Fat 15.7 g
- Saturated Fat 1.7 g
- Carbohydrate 16.9 g
- Dietary Fiber 5.6 g
- Sugars 9.1g Protein 6.8 g

36. Grilled Cauliflower Steak

Preparation time: 10 minutes
Cooking time: 22 minutes
Servings: 2
Ingredients:

- ½ head cauliflower, sliced into 4 thick slices
- 2 tablespoons lemon juice
- 1 tablespoon olive oil
- Sea salt, to taste

Romesco sauce:

- 1/2 cup roasted red peppers, thinly sliced
- 1/4 cup almonds, slivered
- 1/2 large tomato, chopped
- 1/4 teaspoon cumin ground
- 1 teaspoon garlic, minced - 1/4 teaspoon sea salt
- 1/2 tablespoon fresh lemon juice
- Parsley, for garnish

Direction:

1. Set the oven's temperature to 350 degrees F to preheat.
2. Take a small-sized baking sheet and spread the almonds in it.
3. Transfer the almonds in the baking sheet to the oven and roast them for 5 minutes, then immediately remove from the oven. Spread the cauliflower steaks on the cutting board.
4. Thoroughly whisk the lemon juice with oil in a small-sized bowl and rub half of this mixture over the cauliflower steaks. Drizzle some salt on top of the cauliflower steaks.
5. Prepare a grill and let it heat on medium temperature.
6. Grease the grilling grates with cooking spray.
7. Place the seasoned cauliflower steaks in the grill and cook for about 9 minutes until they are soft. Flip the steaks using a tong and brush the remaining oil mixture on top.
8. Cook for another 8 minutes in the grill. Meanwhile, add tomato to a small food processor and hit the pulse button to blend it. Add remaining sauce ingredients to the processor along with toasted almonds. Blend the sauce again into a creamy and smooth mixture.
9. Transfer the grilled cauliflower steaks to the serving plates.
10. Pour the almond sauce over the grilled cauliflower steaks.
11. Garnish with parsley. Serve the sauce over the cauliflower and garnish with parsley.

Nutrition:

- Calories 188 Total Fat 13.4 g Sodium 389mg Carbohydrate 14.9g Dietary Fiber 6g
- Sugars 7.2 g Protein 6.2 g

37. Broccoli Fried Rice

Preparation time: 15 minutes
Cooking time: 15 minutes
Servings: 2
Ingredients:

- 3 cups broccoli, chopped
- 2 teaspoons sesame oil
- 1 small red pepper, chopped
- 1/2 cup carrots, shredded
- 1/3 cup peas, fresh
- 1 small garlic clove, grated
- 1/2 teaspoon fresh ginger, grated
- 2 tablespoons soy sauce
- 1/3 cup green onion, diced

Direction:

1. Cut the broccoli head into small florets.
2. Transfer the broccoli florets to the food processor and hit the pulse button.
3. Grind the broccoli florets for 20 seconds until they form a rice-like texture.
4. Take a large skillet and place it over medium heat.
5. Add sesame oil, carrots, red pepper and peas to the skillet.
6. Stir-fry the veggies for 5 minutes until they are soft and tender.
7. Toss in riced broccoli, soy sauce, garlic, and ginger.
8. Cook the broccoli for 10 minutes with constant stirring.
9. Transfer the broccoli rice to the serving plate.
10. Garnish with green onion and serve.
11. Enjoy.

Nutrition:

- Calories 135
- Total Fat 5.7 g
- Saturated Fat 0. 7g
- Carbohydrate 17.9 g
- Dietary Fiber 6.6 g
- Sugars 6.2 g
- Protein 4.9 g

38. Zucchini Green Bean soup

Preparation time: 20 minutes
Cooking time: 35 minutes
Servings: 2
Ingredients:

- 2 tablespoons olive oil
- 2 onions, chopped
- 1/2 cup celery, chopped
- 2 medium-sized carrots, peeled and chopped
- cloves garlic, finely chopped
- 2 zucchinis, chopped
- oz. fresh green beans, sliced
- oz. cauliflower florets
- 4 cups cabbage leaves, washed and chopped
- 2 quarts low-sodium beef stock
- 2 teaspoons beef bouillon powder
- 1 teaspoon cayenne pepper
- 1 teaspoon salt
- 1/2 teaspoon ground black pepper
- 4 cups packed spinach leaves
- 1/4 cup fresh parsley, chopped
- 2 teaspoons lemon juice

Direction:

1. Take a large-sized stockpot and place it over medium-low heat.
2. Add olive oil to the stockpot and heat it. Stir in celery, carrots, and onions then sauté for 8 minutes until soft.
3. Add garlic and stir-fry for 30 seconds, then toss in green beans and zucchini.
4. Sauté for about 5 minutes or more until the zucchinis are soft, stirring occasionally.
5. Toss cabbage leaves and cauliflower into the stockpot. Pour in the stock and cook the soup to a simmer on high heat. Stir in cayenne and bouillon along with salt and black pepper for seasoning. Reduce the heat of the soup and cook for 20 minutes. Finally, add spinach leaves and cook until they are wilted.
6. Remove the soup from the heat and add lemon juice and parsley.
7. Serve warm and fresh.

Nutrition:

- Calories 180 Total Fat 7. 8g Saturated Fat 1.2 g Carbohydrate 25.8 g Dietary Fiber 9.4 g
- Sugars 11.3 g Protein 6.4 g

39. Mexican Cabbage Soup

Preparation time: 20 minutes
Cooking time: 30 minutes
Servings: 2
Ingredients:

- 1 lb. lean ground beef
- 1/2 teaspoon salt
- 3/4 teaspoon garlic powder
- 1/4 teaspoon black pepper
- 1 tablespoon olive oil
- 1 medium onion, chopped
- 3 cups cabbage, chopped
- 3 cans (4 oz.) green chilis, chopped
- 2 cups water
- 1 can (14-1/2 oz.) low-sodium beef broth
- 2 tablespoons fresh cilantro, minced
- Pico de Gallo, to garnish
- Low-fat sour cream, to garnish

Direction:

1. Take a large-sized saucepan and place it over medium-high heat.
2. Add ½ tbsp olive oil and beef to the saucepan and stir cook for 7 minutes until it turns brown.
3. Transfer the cooked beef to a plate and keep it covered and warm.
4. Add the rest of the olive oil to the same pan and heat it over medium-high heat.
5. Toss in cabbage and onion then sauté for 6 minutes.
6. Once the veggies are soft, return the beef to the pan.
7. Pour in broth and water, then cook the soup to a boil.
8. 8. Add green chillies, garlic powder, black pepper and salt for seasoning.
9. 9. Lower the heat to a simmer and cook the soup on this heat for 10 minutes.
11. Garnish the soup with cilantro, Pico de Gallo and sour cream.
12. Serve warm and fresh.
13. Enjoy.

Nutrition:

- Calories 208 Total Fat 10 g
- Saturated Fat 3.5 g Carbohydrate 7.3 g
- Dietary Fiber 2.2 g Sugars 3.8g Protein 21.1 g

40. Thai Shrimp Soup

Preparation time: 25 minutes
Cooking time: 45 minutes
Servings: 2
Ingredients:

- 1 lb. shrimps, peeled and deveined
- 2 tablespoons coconut oil
- 1 medium onion, diced - 4 garlic cloves, minced
- 1-inch piece ginger root, peeled and sliced
- 1 lemongrass stalk, chopped
- 3 fresh kaffir lime leaves, chopped
- 1 red and 1 green Thai chilies, chopped
- cups chicken broth
- 1/2 lb. shiitake mushrooms, washed and sliced
- 1 small green zucchini, sliced
- 2 tablespoons fresh lime juice - 2 tablespoons fish sauce
- 1/4 bunch fresh cilantro, chopped
- 1/4 bunch fresh Thai basil, chopped
- Salt and black pepper, to taste

Direction:

1. Wash the shrimps and pat them dry. Peel the shrimps and keep their shells aside.
2. Devein the peeled shrimps and keep them on a separate plate.
3. Take a large-sized pot and place it over medium heat.
4. Add coconut oil to the pan and let it heat for a few seconds.
5. Toss in shrimp shells first and stir-fry until they turn red in color.
6. Stir in garlic, ginger, onion, lime leaf, salt, chilies, black pepper, and lemongrass.
12. Sauté the veggies for 3 minutes until onions are soft. Pour in chicken broth and cook the soup to a simmer. Cook the soup for about 30 minutes on this heat and then strain it to discard the shells and the veggies. Return the soup to low heat and keep it warm.
13. Meanwhile, take a large soup pan and place it over high heat.
14. Add zucchini, coconut oil and mushrooms along with salt and black pepper for seasoning.
15. Sauté for 5 minutes then pour in the shrimp broth. Add raw shrimp and cook for 2 minutes until shrimps turn pink. Stir in fish sauce and lime juice. Garnish with fresh cilantro. Serve warm.

Nutrition:

- Calories 197 Total Fat 7.1g Saturated Fat 4.7g Carbohydrate 10.4g Dietary Fiber 1.4g
- Sugars 3.3g Protein 22.7g

41. Beef & Barley Soup

Preparation Time: 10 min.
Cooking Time: 50 min.
Servings: 2
Ingredients:
- ½ c. parsley, finely chopped
- ½ tsp. thyme, dried
- 1 c. wheat barley, hulled
- 1 lb. ground beef
- 1 lg. onion, diced
- 1 tbsp. extra virgin olive oil
- 1 tsp. salt
- 2 lg. stalks celery, diced
- 3 bay leaves
- 3 cloves garlic, minced
- 3 lg. carrots, diced
- 9 c. low-sodium beef broth
- Ground black pepper, to taste

Direction:
1. Heat a large pot or Dutch oven over medium heat and add oil to it.
2. Once the oil is hot, stir the onion and garlic in, allowing them to cook for about three minutes, stirring often.
3. Stir carrots, beef, celery, and thyme into the pot. Brown the beef, breaking it into smaller chunks as you do so.
4. Once the beef is browned, add the broth, salt, pepper, and bay leaves to the pot, stirring completely. Cover the pot and bring to a boil.
5. Once boiling, reduce the heat to low and let simmer for 40 minutes.
6. Remove the pot from the heat and stir, adding the parsley and adjusting the seasoning to suit your taste. Remove the bay leaves and stir once more.
7. Serve hot!

Nutrition:
- Calories: 189
- Carbohydrates: 22 g
- Fat: 4 g
- Protein: 16 g
- Sugar: 3 g

42. Instant Pot Chicken

Preparation Time: 5 min.
Cooking Time: 20 min.
Servings: 2
Ingredients:

- 1 c. water
- 1 tsp. rosemary, chopped
- 1 med. lemon, sliced
- 2 cloves garlic, minced
- 2 lb. chicken thighs, boneless & skinless
- 2 tbsp. extra virgin olive oil
- Sea salt & pepper, to taste

Direction:

1. Combine all ingredients in a medium mixing bowl, incorporate fully and cover.
2. Plug in your Instant Pot and select the Sauté setting. Drizzle a little extra olive oil into the bottom of it to prevent sticking.
3. Once the pot is hot, place the thighs in one even layer on the bottom of the Instant Pot and allow to cook until a golden crust is formed on the chick (about four to five minutes, then flip and allow the other side to cook as well.
4. Pull the thighs out of the pot and use the water to deglaze the bottom of the pot, scraping lightly with your spatula or spoon as you stir the water around the pot.
5. Place the chicken into the pot (on top of the trivet insert if you have one, but no problem if you don't) and place the lid on top. Cook at high pressure for five minutes to cook the chicken the rest of the way through.
6. Release the pressure and remove the chicken from the pot.
7. Serve hot with your favorite sides!

Nutrition:

- Calories: 223
- Carbohydrates: 0 g
- Fat: 11 g
- Protein: 30 g
- Sugar: 0 g

43. Shrimp Salad

Preparation Time: 15 min.

Cooking Time: 0 min.

Servings: 2

Ingredients:
- 1/3 English cucumber, diced
- ¾ c. plain yogurt
- 1 lb. shrimp, cooked & chopped
- 1 tbsp. Dijon mustard
- 1 tsp. garlic powder
- 2 tbsp. mayo
- 3 med. stalks celery, diced
- Sea salt & pepper, to taste

Direction:
1. In a large mixing bowl, combine all ingredients and stir to combine thoroughly.
2. Cover and chill for at least 15 minutes before serving.
3. Serve chilled!

Nutrition:
- Calories: 112
- Carbohydrates: 4 g
- Fat: 5g
- Protein: 14 g
- Sugar: 3 g

44. roccoli Salad

Preparation Time: 20 min.
Cooking Time: 5 min.
Servings: 2
Ingredients:
- ½ c. dried cranberries, unsweetened
- ½ c. pecans, chopped
- ½ c. sunflower seeds
- 1 ½ tbsp. onion powder
- 1 c. plain yogurt
- 1 lb. broccoli, chopped
- 1 sm. bell pepper, diced
- 1 tbsp. apple cider vinegar
- Red pepper flakes, to taste
- Sea salt & pepper, to taste

Direction:
1. In a large mixing bowl, combine all ingredients and stir to combine thoroughly.
2. Cover and chill for at least 15 minutes before serving.
3. Serve chilled!

Nutrition:
- Calories: 234
- Carbohydrates: 20 g
- Fat: 13 g
- Protein: 9 g
- Sugar: 9 g

45. Southwest Chicken Salad

Preparation Time: 15 min.
Cooking Time: 15 min.
Servings: 2
Ingredients:
- ¼ c. extra virgin olive oil
- ¼ c. red onion, finely chopped
- 1 c. corn, drained
- 1 can low-sodium black beans, rinsed & drained
- 1 jalapeño, seeded & minced
- 1 tsp. chili powder
- 1 tsp. cumin
- 1 tsp. garlic powder
- 1 tsp. onion powder
- 2 bell peppers, diced
- 2 lg. limes, juiced
- 2 lb. chicken thighs, cooked and diced
- 2 tbsp. cilantro, finely chopped
- 3 c. quinoa, cooked to package instructions (still hot)
- Sea salt & black pepper, to taste

Direction:
1. In a small bowl, combine lime juice, chili powder, onion powder, garlic powder, cumin, and cilantro. Mix thoroughly and set aside.
2. In a large mixing bowl, combine all other ingredients and toss until thoroughly combined.
3. Drizzle seasoning mixture over the salad and toss to coat completely.
4. Cover and chill for at least 30 minutes.
5. Serve chilled!

Nutrition:
- Calories: 217
- Carbohydrates: 30 g
- Fat: 9 g
- Protein: 7 g
- Sugar: 2 g

46. Tuna Salad

Preparation Time: 15 min.
Cooking Time: 0 min.
Servings: 2
Ingredients:
- ¼ c. mayonnaise
- ¼ c. red onion, finely diced
- ¾ c. plain yogurt
- 1 clove garlic, minced
- 1 lg. stalk celery, diced
- 1 tbsp. lemon juice
- 2 sm. dill pickles, diced
- 24 oz. tuna packed in water, drained
- Sea salt & pepper, to taste

Direction:
1. In a large mixing bowl, combine all ingredients and stir to combine thoroughly.
2. Cover and chill for at least 15 minutes before serving.
3. Serve chilled!

Nutrition:
- Calories: 152
- Carbohydrates: 2 g
- Fat: 8 g
- Protein: 18 g
- Sugar: 1 g

47. Black Bean & Quinoa Salad

Preparation Time: 15 min.
Cooking Time: 15 min.
Servings: 2
Ingredients:

- 3 c. quinoa, cooked to package instructions and cooled
- 14 oz. low-sodium black beans, rinsed and drained
- 1 lg. tomatoes, diced
- 2 tbsp. cilantro, finely chopped
- ¼ c. red onion, finely diced
- 1 jalapeño, seeded & minced
- 1 clove garlic, minced
- 2 lg. limes, juiced
- ¼ c. extra virgin olive oil
- 1 tsp. cumin
- 1 tsp. chili powder
- 1 tsp. onion powder
- Sea salt & pepper to taste

Direction:

1. In a small bowl, combine olive oil, lime juice, cumin, cilantro, salt, pepper, chili powder, and onion powder. Mix thoroughly.
2. In a large mixing bowl, combine all remaining ingredients and stir to combine thoroughly.
3. Drizzle dressing over the mixture and stir once more to combine.
4. Cover and chill for at least 15 minutes before serving.
5. Serve chilled!

Nutrition:

- Calories: 408
- Carbohydrates: 53 g
- Fat: 17 g
- Protein: 14 g
- Sugar: 4 g

48. Pasta Salad

Preparation Time: 8 min.
Cooking Time: 10 min.
Servings: 2
Ingredients:

- 1/8 tsp. red pepper flakes
- 1/3 c. extra virgin olive oil
- 1/3 c. parsley, finely chopped
- ½ c. feta cheese crumbles
- 1 c. Kalamata olives pitted and halved
- 1 lb. fresh green beans, chopped
- 1 tbsp. oregano
- 2 tsp. garlic powder
- 4 sm. tomatoes, diced
- 8 oz. whole-grain macaroni, cooked al dente and cooled
- Sea salt & pepper to taste

Direction:

1. Place chopped green beans into a small pot of water and heat over medium, salting lightly. Stir frequently until the green beans deepen in color, but retain their crisp.
2. Remove the beans from heat and plunge into an ice bath to halt cooking.
3. In a small bowl, combine olive oil, parsley, garlic powder, salt, pepper, oregano, and pepper flakes. Stir to combine thoroughly.
4. In a large mixing bowl, combine all remaining ingredients and mix completely.
5. Drizzle dressing over the mixture and stir once more to coat.
6. Cover and chill for at least 15 minutes before serving.
7. Serve chilled!

Nutrition:

- Calories: 247
- Carbohydrates: 26 g
- Fat: 15 g
- Protein: 7 g
- Sugar: 3 g

49. Thai-Inspired Chicken Salad

Preparation Time: 10 min.
Cooking Time: 0 min.
Servings: 2
Ingredients:

- ¼ c. cilantro, finely chopped
- ¼ c. green onion, chopped
- ½ peanuts, roasted & unsalted
- ½ tsp. red pepper flakes
- 1 c. plain yogurt
- 1 med. bell pepper, diced
- 2 c. red cabbage, chopped
- 2 chicken breasts, cooked and shredded
- 2 tbsp. maple syrup
- 3 tbsp. rice wine vinegar
- Sea salt & pepper to taste

Direction:

1. In a large mixing bowl, combine all ingredients and stir to combine thoroughly.
2. Cover and chill for at least 15 minutes before serving.
3. Serve chilled!

Nutrition:

- Calories: 152
- Carbohydrates: 2 g
- Fat: 8 g
- Protein: 18 g
- Sugar: 1 g

50. Greek Quinoa Salad

Preparation Time: 10 min.

Cooking Time: 15 min.

Servings: 2

Ingredients:
- ¼ c. red onion, finely chopped
- ½ c. feta cheese crumbles
- ½ c. parsley, finely chopped
- ½ English cucumber, chopped
- 1 c. quinoa, cooked according to package instructions and cooled
- 1 lemon, juiced
- 1 lg. bell pepper, chopped
- 1 med. tomato, diced
- 1 tbsp. cumin
- 2 tbsp. extra virgin olive oil
- 20 Kalamata olives pitted and halved
- Sea salt & pepper, to taste

Direction:
1. In a large mixing bowl, combine all ingredients and stir to combine thoroughly.
2. Cover and chill for at least 15 minutes before serving.
3. Serve chilled!

Nutrition:
- Calories: 144
- Carbohydrates: 28 g
- Fat: 23 g
- Protein: 8 g
- Sugar: 3 g

CHAPTER 24:

Dinner

51. Instant Pot Teriyaki Chicken

Preparation Time: 5 minutes
Cooking Time: 35 minutes
Servings: 15
Ingredients
- 1/2 cup soy sauce
- 1/2 cup water
- 1/2 cup brown sugar
- 2 tbsps. rice wine vinegar
- 1 tbsp. mirin (Japanese sweet wine)
- 1 tbsp. sake
- 1 tbsp. minced garlic
- 1 dash freshly cracked black pepper
- 1 lb. skinless, boneless chicken

Directions
1. Combine soy sauce, brown sugar, water, rice wine vinegar, sake, mirin, pepper, and garlic in a bowl to prepare the sauce.
2. Put chicken in an electric pressure cooker (such as Instant Pot(R)). Pour the sauce over.
3. Close lid and lock. Set to Meat function, with the timer on to 12 minutes. Give 10-15 minutes for pressure to build.
4. Gently release pressure with the quick-release method according to manufacturer's instructions, for 5 minutes. Remove lid. Insert the instant read thermometer into the middle of the chicken and make sure to reach at least 165°F (74°C). If not hot enough, cook for 2-4 more minutes.
5. Take chicken out from the cooker. Shred or cut up. Mix with sauce from the pot.

Nutrition:
- Calories: 259 Carbohydrates: 33.1 g
- Protein: 24.3 g
- Fat: 2.3g Sugar: 1 g
- Sodium: 486 mg Fiber: 0 g

52. Teriyaki Salmon

Preparation Time: 15 minutes
Cooking Time: 5 minutes
Servings: 2
Ingredients:
- 3 tbsps. lime juice
- 2 tbsps. olive oil
- 2 tbsps. reduced-sodium teriyaki sauce
- 1 tbsp. balsamic vinegar
- 1 tbsp. Dijon mustard
- 1 tsp. garlic powder
- 6 drops hot pepper sauce
- 6 uncooked jumbo salmon

Directions
1. Mix the first 7 ingredients together in a big zip lock plastic bag then put in the shrimp. Seal the zip lock bag and turn to coat the salmon. Keep in the fridge for an hour and occasionally turn.
2. Drain the marinated salmon and discard marinade. Broil the salmon 4 inches from heat for 3 to 4 minutes per side or until the salmon turn pink in color.

Nutrition:
- Calories: 93
- Carbohydrates: 3 g
- Protein: 13 g
- Fat: 4 g
- Sugar: 1.6 g
- Sodium: 176 mg
- Fiber: 0 g

53. Sheet Pan Steak Fajitas

Preparation Time: 5 minutes
Cooking Time: 8 minutes
Servings: 15
Ingredients:

- 1 pound of flank steak, sliced into strips
- 1 tablespoon of taco seasoning
- 1 (16-ounce) bag of frozen onion and peppers slices
- 1 (15-ounce) Can have diced tomatoes with green chiles
- ¼ cup of homemade low-sodium beef broth
- 1 bunch of fresh cilantros, chopped
- 2 medium lime, juice and zest
- Fine sea salt and freshly cracked black pepper (to taste)

Directions

1. Add all the ingredients except for the lime juice and lime zest inside your Instant Pot. Lock the lid and cook at high pressure for 8 minutes.
2. When the cooking is done, naturally release the pressure and carefully remove the lid.
3. Stir in the lime juice and lime zest. Top the fajitas onto cauliflower rice or lettuce leaves. Serve and enjoy!

Nutrition:

- Calories: 49
- Carbohydrates: 7 g
- Protein: 15 g
- Fat: 3 g
- Sugar: 0 g
- Sodium: 180 mg
- Fiber: 0 g

54. Instant Pot Meatballs

Preparation Time: 5 minutes
Cooking Time: 30 minutes
Servings: 4
Ingredients:
- 2 pounds of ground meat
- 1 small onion, finely chopped
- 4 medium garlic cloves, peeled and minced
- 2 large organic eggs
- 4 tablespoons of ranch dressing
- 4 tablespoons of almond flour
- 2 tablespoons of fresh parsley, finely chopped
- 2 tablespoons of Worcestershire sauce
- 1 cup of Frank's Buffalo Hot Sauce
- ½ cup of unsalted butter
- ½ cup of water

Directions
1. In a large bowl, add the ground meat, onion, garlic, eggs, ranch dressing, parsley, and almond flour. Mix until well combined.
2. Preheat your broiler. Form into meatballs and place onto a baking sheet. Broil for 10 minutes or until brown. Remove and set aside.
3. Press the "Sauté" function on your Instant Pot and add the butter. Once melted, stir in the hot sauce, Worcestershire sauce and water.
4. Stir in the chicken meatballs and lock the lid. Cook at high pressure for 15 minutes. When the cooking is done, naturally release the pressure for 10 minutes, then quick release the remaining pressure. Carefully remove the lid. Serve and enjoy!

Nutrition:
- Calories: 103
- Carbohydrates: 3 g
- Protein: 19 g
- Fat: 4 g
- Sugar: 0.6 g
- Sodium: 908 mg
- Fiber: 0 g

55. Sheet Pan Chicken and Veggie Bake

Preparation Time: 10 minutes
Cooking Time: 50 minutes
Servings: 6

Ingredients

- 2 pounds red potatoes (about 6 medium), cut into 3/4-inch pieces
- 1 large onion, coarsely chopped
- 2 tablespoons olive oil
- 3 garlic cloves, minced
- 1-1/4 teaspoons salt, divided
- 1 teaspoon dried rosemary, crushed, divided
- 3/4 teaspoon pepper, divided
- 1/2 teaspoon paprika
- 6 bone-in chicken thighs (about 2-1/4 pounds), skin removed
- 6 cups fresh baby spinach (about 6 ounces)

Directions

1. Preheat oven to 425°. In a large bowl, combine potatoes, onion, oil, garlic, 3/4 teaspoon salt, 1/2 teaspoon rosemary and 1/2 teaspoon pepper; toss to coat. Transfer to a 15x10x1-in. baking pan coated with cooking spray.
2. In a small bowl, mix paprika and the remaining salt, rosemary and pepper. Sprinkle chicken with paprika mixture; arrange over vegetables. Roast until a thermometer inserted in chicken reads 170°-175° and vegetables are just tender, 35-40 minutes.
3. Remove chicken to a serving platter; keep warm. Top vegetables with spinach. Roast until vegetables are tender and spinach is wilted, 8-10 minutes longer. Stir vegetables to combine; serve with chicken.

Nutrition:

- Calories: 87
- Carbohydrates: 79.03 g
- Protein: 70.74 g
- Fat: 53.13 g
- Sugar: 7.2 g
- Sodium: 2019 mg
- Fiber: 10.3 g

56. Quinoa and Black Bean Casserole

Preparation Time: 10 minutes
Cooking Time: 50 minutes
Servings: 7
Ingredients
- 2 tablespoons canola oil
- 1 medium onion, minced
- 1 tablespoon minced jalapeño pepper
- 2 garlic cloves, minced
- ¼ teaspoon salt
- 1 cup quinoa
- 1½ cups low-sodium chicken broth
- 1 (14.5-ounce) can diced tomatoes, drained
- 1 (14.5-ounce) can black beans, rinsed and drained
- ½ cup grated pepper jack cheese
- ¼ cup chopped cilantro
- 2 scallions, trimmed and thinly sliced

Directions
1. Preheat the oven to 350º F and spray a 9 × 9 casserole dish lightly with nonstick spray.
2. Heat the oil in a medium saucepan over medium-high heat. When hot, add the onion, jalapeño, garlic, and salt. Cook, stirring often, until the vegetables are slightly softened, about 4 minutes.
3. Stir in the quinoa and chicken broth, then bring the mixture to a boil. Gently stir in the tomatoes, black beans, and pepper jack cheese; pour the mixture into the prepared casserole dish.
3. Bake, covered, until the quinoa is cooked through and the vegetables are tender, about 45 minutes.
4. Stir the cilantro and scallions into the casserole just before serving.

Nutrition:
- Calories: 72
- Carbohydrates: 12g
- Protein: 18g
- Fat: 8.3g
- Sugar: 1.4g
- Sodium: 402mg
- Fiber: 13g

57. Haddock with Spinach and Cauliflower Rice

Preparation Time: 10 minutes
Cooking Time: 5 minutes
Servings: 6
Ingredients:
- 1 pound of haddock fillets, frozen
- 2 cups of frozen spinach
- 2 tablespoons of extra-virgin olive oil
- 1 teaspoon of fine sea salt
- 1 teaspoon of freshly cracked black pepper
- 2 cups of cauliflower rice
- Lemon Garlic Mayonnaise Ingredients:
- 2 tablespoons of mayonnaise
- 2 teaspoons of freshly squeezed lemon juice
- 1 teaspoon of minced garlic

Directions
1. In a small bowl, add the mayonnaise, lemon juice and garlic. Stir well and set aside.
2. Add 1 cup of water and a trivet inside your Instant Pot.
3. In a heat-safe dish that fits inside your Instant Pot, add the cauliflower rice and spinach. Place the haddock fillets on top.
4. Season the haddock fillets with sea salt and black pepper. Drizzle with olive oil.
5. Place the dish on top of the trivet and lock the lid.
6. Cook at high pressure for 6 minutes. When the cooking is done, quick release the pressure and remove the lid. Serve and enjoy!

Nutrition:
- Calories: 115
- Carbohydrates: 5 g
- Protein: 25 g
- Fat: 12 g
- Sugar: 0 g
- Sodium: 645 mg
- Fiber: 0 g

58. Zoodles with White Clam Sauce

Preparation Time: 5 minutes
Cooking Time: 15 minutes
Servings: 7
Ingredients:
- 2 pounds of small clams
- 3 large zucchinis, spiralized
- ¼ cup of unsalted butter
- 2 tablespoons of extra-virgin olive oil
- 1 tablespoon of garlic, minced
- ½ cup of dry white wine
- 2 tablespoons of freshly squeezed lemon juice
- 1 teaspoon of lemon zest
- 1 teaspoon of fine sea salt
- ¼ teaspoon of freshly cracked black pepper
- ¼ cup of fresh parsley, finely chopped

Directions
1. Press the "Sauté" setting on your Instant Pot and add the olive oil and butter. Once hot, add the minced garlic and sauté for 2 minutes or until fragrant, stirring frequently.
2. Add the dry white wine and lemon juice. Cook for 2 minutes or until most of the liquid evaporates, stirring frequently.
3. Add the clams and cook for 3 minutes or until the clams has opened up.
4. Turn off the "Sauté" setting on your Instant Pot and stir in the spiralized zucchini. Stir until well coated with liquid.
5. Stir in the lemon zest and fresh parsley. Season with sea salt and freshly cracked black pepper.
6. Serve and enjoy!

Nutrition:
- Calories: 71
- Carbohydrates: 7 g
- Protein: 12 g
- Fat: 4 g
- Sugar: 0.7 g
- Sodium: 219 mg
- Fiber: 0 g

59. Creamy Lamb Korma

Preparation Time: 5 minutes
Cooking Time: 35 minutes
Servings: 9
Ingredients:

- 1 pound of lamb steak, cut into 1-inch pieces
- 1 tablespoon of extra-virgin olive oil
- 1 medium onion, finely chopped
- 1-inch piece of ginger, peeled and minced
- 6 medium garlic cloves, peeled and minced
- 2 tablespoons of tomato paste
- ½ cup of coconut milk or plain yogurt
- ¾ cups of water
- 3 teaspoons of garam masala
- ½ teaspoon of turmeric powder
- 1 teaspoon of smoked or regular paprika
- ½ teaspoon of cardamom powder
- Fine sea salt and freshly cracked black pepper (to taste)

Directions

1. Press the "Sauté" setting on your Instant Pot and add the olive oil. Once hot, add the chopped onions, minced garlic and minced ginger. Sauté for 1 minutes, stirring frequently.
2. Add the tomato paste along with ¼ cup of water. Give a good stir.
3. Stir in all the seasonings and give another good stir.
4. Stir in the coconut milk, the remainder of the water and lamb pieces. Lock the lid and cook at high pressure for 15 minutes. When the cooking is done, naturally release the pressure and remove the lid.
5. Serve and enjoy!

Nutrition:

- Calories: 80
- Carbohydrates: 5 g
- Protein: 26 g
- Fat: 25 g
- Sugar: 0 g
- Sodium: 564 mg
- Fiber: 0 g

60. Fire-Roasted Tomato and Garlic Soup

Preparation Time: 5 minutes
Cooking Time: 10 minutes
Servings: 2
Ingredients:

- 4 (14.5-ounce) cans of fire-roasted tomatoes, undrained
- 8 garlic cloves, peeled and crushed
- 2 tablespoons of extra-virgin olive oil
- 2 cups of homemade low-sodium chicken stock
- Fine sea salt and freshly cracked black pepper (to taste)

Directions

1. Press the "Sauté" setting on your Instant Pot and add the olive oil. Once hot, add the crushed garlic and sauté for 1 minute or until fragrant. Be careful not to overcook the garlic.
2. Add the remaining ingredients and lock the lid. Cook at high pressure for 8 minutes. When the cooking is done naturally release the pressure and remove the lid.
3. Stir the soup again and adjust the seasoning if necessary. If you want, use an immersion blender to puree the soup until smooth. Serve and enjoy!

Nutrition:

- Calories: 121
- Carbohydrates: 5 g
- Protein: 12 g
- Fat: 6 g
- Sugar: 0 g
- Sodium: 432 mg
- Fiber: 0 g

61. Chicken and Prosciutto Spiedini

Preparation Time: 15 minutes
Cooking Time: 10 minutes
Servings: 2
Ingredients:

- raw chicken tenders
- oz. block provolone cheese
- 8 slices prosciutto
- ½ tsp kosher salt
- 1/8 Tsp ground black pepper
- 16 fresh basil leaves
- ¼ tsp garlic powder
- 8 skewers

Directions:

1. Combine the garlic powder, kosher salt, and pepper.
2. Trim the chicken tenders of the tendons, and then pound them out to a half-inch thickness.
3. Season the chicken with the spice mixture.
4. Cut the provolone cheese into pieces about 1-2 inches long.
5. On a cutting board, place a slice of prosciutto. Then top with a chicken tender and two leaves of fresh basil. Next place a piece of cheese across the basil.
6. Carefully roll the bundle and skewer it.
7. Preheat a grill to 325-375°F. Grill for about 3-5 minutes per side, or until a thermometer reads 165°F in the center and the skewers are cooked through.
8. Serve warm.

Nutrition:

- Carbohydrates: 0.75 g
- Fat: 10 g
- Protein: 20 g
- Calories: 174

62. Pinchos de Pollo Marinated Grilled Chicken Kebabs

Preparation Time: 10 minutes (+2 hours)
Cooking Time: 10 minutes
Servings: 2
Ingredients:
- 1½ lb. boneless, skinless chicken breast
- 1 tbsp. minced garlic
- ½ tsp fine Himalayan salt
- ½ tsp freshly ground black pepper
- 1 tsp dried oregano
- 1 tbsp. extra-virgin olive oil
- Juice of one lime
- 7-9 skewers

Directions:
1. Have ready 7-9 soaked skewers.
2. In a bowl, combine the salt, garlic, pepper, lime juice, oregano, and oil.
3. Cut chicken breast into 1-inch chunks and place in a container with a lid.
4. Pour the marinade over the chicken and stir. Cover and refrigerate at least for 2 hours or overnight.
5. Preheat a grill to 325-375°F.
6. Remove the chicken from the refrigerator and thread onto the skewers, leaving a very small space between each piece and spreading each piece as flat as possible.
7. Once the grill is hot, grill the kebabs over direct medium heat, about 8-10 minutes total, keeping the lid closed until the chicken is no longer pink in the center and firm to the touch, turning once or twice during cooking. Take care not overcook.
8. Remove from the grill and serve immediately!

Nutrition:
- Carbohydrates: 3 g
- Fat: 10 g
- Protein: 9 g
- Calories: 290

63. Slow Cooker Bacon and Chicken

Preparation Time: 5 minutes
Cooking Time: 8 hours
Servings: 4
Ingredients:

- chicken breasts
- slices bacon
- 2 tbsp. thyme, dried
- 1 tbsp. oregano, dried
- 1 tbsp. rosemary, dried
- tbsp. olive oil, divided
- 1 tbsp. salt

Directions:

1. Into a slow cooker pot, combine all the ingredients and two tablespoons of olive oil.
2. Cook on low for 8 hours.
3. Shred the meat and mix with remaining olive oil.

Nutrition:

- Carbohydrates: 3.6 g
- Fat: 24 g
- Protein: 22.9 g
- Calories: 315

64. Garlic Bacon Wrapped Chicken Bites

Preparation Time: 10 minutes
Cooking Time: 30 minutes
Servings: 4
Ingredients:

- 1 large skinless chicken breast, cut into small bites
- slices bacon, cut into thirds
- tbsp. garlic powder

Directions:

1. Preheat the oven to 400°F. Line a baking tray with foil.
2. Place the garlic powder in a bowl and dip each piece of chicken into the garlic powder.
3. Wrap each bacon piece around each garlic chicken bite.
4. Place each bite on the baking tray, spacing them out so that they're not touching.
5. Bake for 25-30 minutes until crispy.

Nutrition:

- Carbohydrates: 5.3 g
- Fat: 5.9 g
- Protein: 23.5 g
- Calories: 170

65. Smokey Bacon Chicken Meatballs

Preparation Time: 15 minutes
Cooking Time: 30 minutes
Servings: 2
Ingredients:

- 1 lb. chicken breasts
- slices bacon, cooked, crumbled
- 1 egg, whisked
- 2 cloves garlic
- 1 tbsp. onion powder
- 2 drops liquid smoke
- tbsps. Olive oil, to cook with
- 2 sprigs fresh parsley, to garnish

Directions:

1. Into a food processor, place all the ingredients except the oil and mix well.
2. Form 20-24 small meatballs from the mixture.
3. Add the oil to a large frying pan, and allow to heat up.
4. Cook meatballs one side for 5 minutes until browned, then flip and cook on the other side for 5-10 minutes until done.
5. Serve immediately!

Nutrition:

- Carbohydrates: 1 g
- Fat: 25 g
- Protein: 13 g
- Calories: 280

66. Asian Chicken Wings

Preparation Time: 10 minutes
Cooking Time: 35 minutes
Servings: 2
Ingredients:
- 2 lbs. chicken wings
- 2 tbsp. sesame oil
- ¼ cup tamari sauce
- 1 tbsp. ginger powder
- 2 tsp white wine vinegar
- cloves garlic, minced
- ¼ tsp sea salt

Directions:
1. Preheat oven to 400°F.
2. In a large container whisk together the ginger powder, sesame oil, salt, tamari sauce, vinegar, and garlic.
3. Add the wings to the mixture and stir to coat.
4. Place the wings on a lined baking sheet and bake for 30-35 minutes until golden and crispy.
5. If you want it crispier, turn on the broiler for a few minutes. Enjoy!

Nutrition:
- Carbohydrates: 1 g
- Fat: 22 g
- Protein: 18 g
- Calories: 277

67. Baked Garlic Ghee Chicken Breast

Preparation Time: 5 minutes
Cooking Time: 30 minutes
Servings: 2
Ingredients:

- 1 chicken breast
- 1 tsp garlic powder
- 1 tbsp. ghee
- 2 cloves garlic, chopped
- 1 tsp sea salt
- 1 tsp chives, diced

Directions:

1. Preheat oven to 350°F.
2. Place the chicken breast on a piece of foil.
3. Season with sea salt, garlic powder, chopped fresh garlic.
4. Top with ghee and rub everything into the chicken breast.
5. Wrap the chicken breast in the foil and place on a baking tray.
6. Bake for 30 minutes, or until chicken breast is cooked through, with a meat thermometer reading above 165°F.
7. Serve with more salt and ghee to taste. Cut the chicken breast into slices and sprinkle diced chives on top.

Nutrition:

- Carbohydrates: 6.1 g
- Fat: 15.5 g
- Protein: 23.7 g
- Calories: 264

68. Crispy Chicken Thighs

Preparation Time: 5 minutes
Cooking Time: 40 minutes
Servings: 2
Ingredients:
- 12 chicken thighs
- tbsps. Olive oil
- 2 tbsps. Salt
- 2 sprigs fresh rosemary, chopped

Directions:
1. Preheat oven to 450° F.
2. Rub salt on each chicken thigh and place on a greased baking tray.
3. Drizzle the olive oil over the chicken thighs and top with the rosemary.
4. Bake for 40 minutes until golden and crispy. Enjoy!

Nutrition:
- Carbohydrates: 0 g
- Fat: 56 g
- Protein: 48 g
- Calories: 713

69. Chicken and Bacon Sausages

Preparation Time: 10 minutes
Cooking Time: 20 minutes
Servings: 2

- Ingredients:
- 1 lb. chicken breasts
- 2 slices bacon, cooked, crumbled
- 1 egg, whisked
- 2 tbsp. Italian seasoning
- 2 tsp garlic powder
- 2 tsp onion powder
- ½ tsp salt
- ½ tsp pepper

Directions:

1. Preheat the oven to 425° F.
2. Put all the ingredients into a food processor and process well.
3. From the meat mixture form approximately 12 thin patties (½-inch thick) and place on a baking tray lined with foil.
4. Bake for 20 minutes, until a meat thermometer shows 170° F.
5. Serve immediately or store in the freezer for 4 weeks.

Nutrition:

- Carbohydrates: 3 g
- Fat: 21 g
- Protein: 40 g
- Calories: 370

70. Bifteck Hache (French Hamburgers)

Preparation Time: 15 minutes
Cooking Time: 20 minutes
Servings: 4
Ingredients:
Burgers
- 1½ lb. ground beef
- tbsps. Ghee
- 1 onion, diced
- 1 egg
- 1 tbsp. fresh thyme leaves
- ½ tsp. salt
- ½ tsp. pepper

Sauce
- ½ cup beef stock
- 2 tbsps. Ghee
- ¼ cup parsley, chopped

Directions:
Burgers
1. Place 2 tbsps. Of ghee into a frying pan and cook half the diced onions until translucent, about 2-3 minutes.
2. Allow the onions to cool and add them with the oil in the pan to a mixing bowl with the egg, ground beef, salt, pepper, and thyme leaves.
3. Mix well and form 8 patties.
4. In a frying pan, cook the patties with 2 tbsps. Of ghee until both sides are well browned, about 5-6 minutes per side.

Sauce
1. Place the ghee into a frying pan and sauté the remaining half of the onions, until translucent, about 2-3 minutes.
2. Add the beef stock and let cook until reduced, about 2-3 minutes. Add in the parsley.
3. Serve the sauce with the burgers.

Nutrition:
- Carbohydrates: 1 g
- Fat: 36 g
- Protein: 35 g
- Calories: 460

71. Lemon Ghee Roast Chicken

Preparation Time: 10 minutes
Cooking Time: 1 hour 45 minutes
Servings: 8
Ingredients:
- lb. whole chicken, remove giblets
- 1 lemon, zested, sliced
- 1 lemon, halved
- ½ cup ghee
- 1 tbsp. salt

Directions:
1. Preheat the oven to 350° F.
2. Combine lemon zest and ½ tbsp. salt and rub all over the chicken.
3. Sprinkle ½ tbsp. salt into the chicken cavity and stuff with lemon halves and ¼ cup of ghee.
4. Brush the remaining ghee on the outside of the chicken.
5. Place the chicken in a roasting pan and arrange the lemon slices around the chicken.
6. Roast for 1 hour 45 minutes. Using a meat thermometer, cook until the internal temperature of the meat is 165°F.
7. Let the chicken rest for about 10 minutes before slicing and serving.

Nutrition:
- Carbohydrates: 0 g
- Fat: 30 g
- Protein: 43 g
- Calories: 91432

72. Oven-Baked Parmesan Garlic Wings

Preparation Time: 5 minutes
Cooking Time: 30 minutes
Servings: 12
Ingredients:
- lbs. whole chicken wings
- tbsp. butter, melted
- 1 egg
- ½ tsp Italian seasoning
- ½ cup Parmesan cheese
- 1 tsp garlic powder
- ¼ tsp crushed red pepper
- ¼ tsp salt

Directions:
1. Preheat the oven to 425° F. cut the wings into two pieces.
2. Put the wings on a baking sheet with a metal rack on top. Cook for 15 minutes.
3. Make the sauce by combining the cheese, butter, seasonings, and egg in a small bowl. Don't worry about using a raw egg in the sauce; the wings will be hot enough.
4. Remove the wings from the oven and flip them over. Turn on the broiler and broil for 5 minutes. Flip again and broil for another 5 minutes. Keep flipping and broiling until they are done to your desired crispness. They should reach an internal temperature of 165°F.
5. Toss immediately in the sauce.
6. Garnish with extra cheese.

Nutrition:
- Carbohydrates: 0.6 g
- Fat: 45.9 g
- Protein: 45.4 g
- Calories: 602

73. Crispy Indian Chicken Drumsticks

Preparation Time: 5 minutes
Cooking Time: 40 minutes
Servings: 5
Ingredients:

- 2 lbs. chicken drumsticks
- 2 tbsps. Salt
- tbsp. garam masala
- ½ tbsp. coconut oil

Directions:

1. Preheat the oven to 450° F
2. Smear a large baking tray with coconut oil.
3. In a bowl, mix the garam masala and salt.
4. Pat the drumsticks dry.
5. Coat each drumstick with the mixture and lay on the baking tray.
6. Bake for 40 minutes. Serve immediately.

Nutrition:

- Carbohydrates: 3.6 g
- Fat: 24.3 g
- Protein: 34.7 g
- Calories: 362

74. Whole Roast Chicken

Preparation Time: 15 minutes
Cooking Time: 1 hour 30 minutes
Servings: 8
Ingredients:
- lbs. whole organic chicken
- 2 sprigs fresh rosemary
- 2 garlic cloves
- 1 tsp Herbes de Provence
- 1 tbsp. coarse sea salt

Directions:
1. Preheat oven to 350°F.
2. Rinse the chicken well under cold water.
3. Place chicken on a baking pan, breast up.
4. Stuff the cavity with the garlic cloves and rosemary.
5. Mix the salt and Herbs the Provence in a small bowl. Sprinkle half of the mixture on the breast.
6. Turn chicken breast side down and sprinkle the remaining mixture on the top.
7. Bake for 1 hour 30 minutes, until the chicken skin is nicely browned.
8. Serve immediately.

Nutrition:
- Carbohydrates: 0.4 g
- Fat: 13.7 g
- Protein: 29.3 g
- Calories: 143

75. Butternut Squash Tacos with Tempeh Chorizo

Preparation Time: 50 minutes
Cooking Time: 10 minutes
Servings: 4
Ingredients:

- One 8-ounce package tempeh
- ½ cup of filtered water
- ¼ cup apple cider vinegar
- 2 cups butternut squash, peeled, cut into cubes
- 1 teaspoon chili powder
- ½ teaspoon smoked paprika
- ½ teaspoon cumin
- ½ teaspoon garlic powder
- ½ teaspoon oregano
- A dash of cayenne
- 1 tablespoon nutritional yeast
- A few dashes of liquid smoke
- Black pepper and sea salt to taste
- ½ cup thinly julienned carrot (optional)
- 8 corn tortillas (or whatever you have on hand)
- 1 large avocado, pitted and sliced
- Cilantro, chopped

Direction

1. Cut the tempeh into two parts. Steam for 10 min. Place in a large bowl and tear apart into small pieces either with your hands (after it's cooled) or with a pastry cutter.
2. While tempeh is steaming, bring water and vinegar to a boil in a small skillet.
3. Add spices, squash, liquid smoke, nutritional yeast, and a pinch of sea salt to skillet. Coat well and simmer covered, stirring occasionally. Add carrots and tempeh, covering again. Simmer a little while longer, stirring to prevent sticking. Uncover and season with pepper and salt.
4. Fill warmed tortillas with squash and tempeh mix and top with avocado and cilantro.

Nutrition:

- Carbohydrates: 45.27 g
- Fat: 15.25 g
- Protein: 16.66 g
- Calories: 357

Conclusion

Intermittent fasting is a great way to maintain a healthy weight, reduce the risk of cancer, and keep your blood sugar in check. There are no risks to women over 50 when it comes to fasting. If you are over 50 and considering fasting, consult your doctor first.

Fasting on a regular basis can be an excellent way for the overweight or obese to lose weight and maintain a healthy weight without resorting to calorie restriction or unhealthy dieting practices.

There are many methods of intermittent fasting, many of which can effectively help people lose weight. A common approach is alternate day-fasting or "EOD" (every other day) which involves eating normally for 24 hours followed by a 24 hour fast. Those who follow the alternate-day fasting scheme can eat their biggest meal on the non-fasting days, or "feast days" which will help them to maintain their energy levels and their calorie intake while also helping them to lose weight.

Another popular method of intermittent fasting is the 5:2 diet. This involves eating normally for five days of the week and restricting your calorie intake to 500-600 calories on two non-consecutive days (the so-called "fasting days"). This method can also be combined with meal timing, such as eating your first meal at noon and your last meal at 7 pm which is a particularly effective way of reducing food cravings and maintaining good energy levels throughout the day.

As well as dieting strategies, periodic fasting helps reduce insulin levels in the body which may reduce the risk of cancer by inhibiting cell growth. In a study, scientists at the University of California analyzed the effects of fasting on breast cancer cells and found that fasting for two days caused cell death in mice, while another research team at the University of Regensburg in Germany found that fasting 16 And 24 hours will greatly reduce insulin levels in mice, thereby reducing the risk of cancer. Also, the cells in a fasting body switch to burning fat instead of carbohydrates which reduces the levels of a substance produced by the body called glucose-6-phosphate. This substance is highly reactive in that it increases the risk for cancer, so its reduction can reduce this risk.

For those who are overweight and considering intermittent fasting to help them lose weight, one of the things they need to consider is how they will feel when they start fasting. If you are used to eating three meals each day and suddenly decide you are going to cut your calories dramatically, it's possible that you'll be hungry most of the time during your first few weeks of fasting. However, this will likely be a temporary state which will pass after a few weeks. Many people find that they do the best when they eat their biggest meal on the non-fasting days and then limit their calorie intake to around 500-600 calories for the rest of the day.

One common concern people have about fasting is how it can affect their blood sugar levels and insulin sensitivity. Some studies have found that intermittent fasting causes a rise in blood sugar levels, but these studies have usually involved adult men who fasted for shorter periods of time than women. For women over 50, fasting does not seem to cause problems with blood sugar as long as you are healthy without pre-existing conditions such as diabetes or hypoglycemia.

The same applies to insulin sensitivity after people have fasted. One study found no negative effects on insulin sensitivity for women who fasted. Another study examined the effect of fasting during Ramadan on the insulin sensitivity and glucose tolerance of healthy men and women (with or without diabetes), who fasted for 16-18 hours a day during the Holy Month. The study found that fasting had no negative effect on blood sugar in women who had healthy blood sugar levels, but those with diabetes experienced an increase in their blood sugar levels.

For both men and women over 50, intermittent fasting is a great way to help reduce weight while improving health. Both men and women can participate in intermittent fasting without risking side effects.

Printed in Great Britain
by Amazon